Visit our

to find out about additional books from Chur
and other Harcourt Health Sciences imprints

Register free at
www.harcourt-international.com

and you will get

- **the latest information on new books, journals and electronic products in your chosen subject areas**

- **the choice of e-mail or post alerts or both, when there are any new books in your chosen areas**

- **news of special offers and promotions**

- **information about products from all Harcourt Health Sciences imprints including Baillière Tindall, Churchill Livingstone, Mosby and W. B. Saunders**

You will also find an easily searchable catalogue, online ordering, information on our extensive list of journals...and much more!

Visit the Harcourt Health Sciences website today!

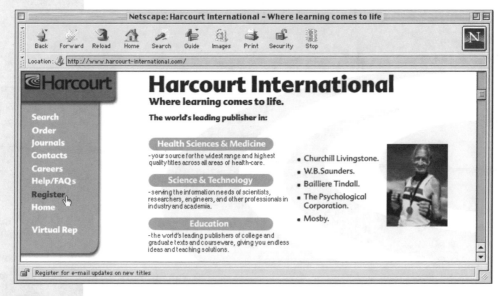

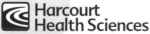

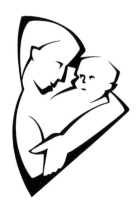

Clinical Aromatherapy for

Pregnancy and Childbirth

For Churchill Livingstone:

Senior Commissioning Editor: Inta Ozols
Project Development Manager: Karen Gilmour
Project Manager: Jane Shanks
Design Direction: George Ajayi

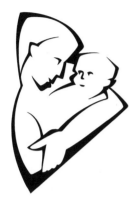

Clinical Aromatherapy for Pregnancy and Childbirth

Denise Tiran RGN RM ADM MTD PGCEA
Principal Lecturer, Complementary Therapies/Midwifery;
Programme Leader – BSc(Hons) Complementary Therapies
School of Health, University of Greenwich, London, UK

SECOND EDITION

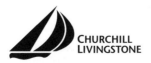

CHURCHILL
LIVINGSTONE

EDINBURGH LONDON NEW YORK PHILADELPHIA ST LOUIS SYDNEY TORONTO 2000

CHURCHILL LIVINGSTONE
An imprint of Harcourt Publishers Limited

© Baillière Tindall 1996
© Harcourt Publishers Limited 2000

 is a registered trademark of Harcourt Publishers Limited

The right of Denise Tiran to be identified as author of this work has been asserted
by her in accordance with the Copyright, Designs and Patents Act 1988

First edition 1996
Second edition 2000

0 443 06427 X

British Library Cataloguing in Publication Data
A catalogue record for this book is available from the British Library

Library of Congress Cataloging in Publication Data
A catalog record for this book is available from the Library of Congress

Note
Medical knowledge is constantly changing. As new information becomes available,
changes in treatment, procedures, equipment and the use of drugs become necessary.
The author and the publishers have taken care to ensure that the information given
in this text is accurate and up to date. However, readers are strongly advised to
confirm that the information, especially with regard to drug usage, complies with
the latest legislation and standards of practice.

The
publisher's
policy is to use
**paper manufactured
from sustainable forests**

Printed in China

Contents

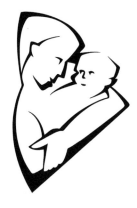

The colour plates are located between pages 118 and 119

Preface

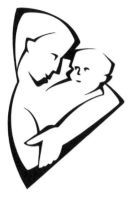

Pregnancy and childbirth are normal, natural, physiological and social events in the lives of many women, their partners and their families, which present exciting challenges and the need for major adaptations. Aromatherapy can act as a complement to the conventional care offered by midwives, medical and other staff, enhancing wellbeing and improving health.

However, while there has been an enormous increase in popularity of the use of essential oils, there has also, quite appropriately, come a note of caution regarding safety and efficacy of these pleasant smelling oils, especially when the client is pregnant. On the one hand women are discouraged from taking any medication that may harm the growing fetus, and on the other they are faced with huge commercial pressure to enjoy a variety of substances about which there initially appears to be little evidence of safety.

The first edition of this book developed as a resource primarily for midwives who may be caring for expectant mothers wishing to self-administer essential oils for pregnancy and labour, or to help them learn more about both the science and the art of utilizing aromatherapy for their clients. The focus was very much on bringing together all the aromatherapy factual and scientific information available at the time, while acknowledging that midwives would already possess adequate maternity-specific knowledge. Later, I became aware that many aromatherapists were keen to specialize in the care of pregnant and labouring women and that they, too, needed additional information to help them provide a safe and satisfying service to the women. However, whereas midwives were required to study aspects of aromatherapy, therapists needed a more in-depth study of maternity physiology, potential pathology and the conventional maternity services than their basic aromatherapy preparation would have provided. This second edition is an attempt to redress the balance by drawing together the relevant theory of both professions in order that each practitioner, whether working in conventional maternity care or in complementary medicine, can be facilitated in offering the safest and most satisfying maternity-related aromatherapy that is possible.

I consider myself to be in an extremely privileged – and unique – position. Having trained as a midwife and worked in the community and later as a midwifery lecturer, I was fortunate enough to become involved in complementary therapies in the late 1980s when the whole field was expanding and facing great change and increased professionalization. For many years now I have been working as a principal lecturer in the School of Health at the University of Greenwich in southeast London, offering a Diploma of Higher Education and a Bachelor of Science honours degree in Complementary Therapies, providing students with an option to study aromatherapy, as well as other therapies. At the same time I have maintained my clinical practice at the nearby maternity unit at Queen Mary's Hospital, Sidcup, in Kent, where I run a complementary therapy service in the antenatal clinic. I use a variety of therapies, including aromatherapy, reflexology, massage, homeopathy, Bach flower remedies, nutrition and elements of Traditional Chinese Medicine (acupuncture, acupressure and moxibustion), to treat a range of problems in pregnancy, labour and the puerperium. The mothers are referred by their midwives, obstetricians or general practitioners, or themselves request information and advice about complementary therapies.

The women who attend the clinic appreciate the time and attention they enjoy from receiving the therapies and also obtain relief from the physiopathological and psychological problems with which they have presented. Many mothers would like longer sessions but this becomes impossible when I am in attendance only one day a week. Thus part of the reason for writing this text is to inform professionals so that they, too, may advocate the value of essential oils in pregnancy and childbirth and take steps towards a greater integration of aromatherapy for their maternity clients.

Over a period of many years I have been honoured to make contact with other professionals keen to integrate complementary therapies into maternity care. This resulted, in 1994, in the founding of the Complementary Therapies in Midwifery National Interest Group, which later evolved into the Complementary Therapies in Maternity Care National Forum, of which I am proud to be the Chair. This is a support network and an educational forum for any health professionals involved in or interested in using complementary therapies during pregnancy and childbearing, which meets three times a year in venues around the country. The interest among midwives has been astounding and gradually we have witnessed an increase in availability of aromatherapy within the maternity services. Similarly the number of aromatherapists wanting to specialize in providing high-quality, evidence-based use of essential oils for pregnant clients has risen. In addition, the incidence of pregnant women requesting advice about aromatherapy from their caregivers has highlighted the need for all professionals to have at least a modicum of knowledge on the subject or to be able to refer women to an appropriately authoritative source of information.

In no way do I infer monopolistic authority on the issue of safe, effective and appropriate administration of essential oils in pregnancy, labour and the puerperium. However, I would like to think that, to some extent, I have succeeded in offering a textbook that presents a comprehensive exploration of this topic, based on evidence from a variety of sources, sufficient to engender a sense of enthusiasm in colleagues that may facilitate a greater expansion of maternity-related aromatherapy. I hope you enjoy reading the results of my work.

London 2000   Denise Tiran

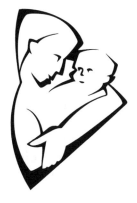

Chapter 1 **Incorporating Aromatherapy into Maternity Care**

Aromatherapy is a science and an art in which highly concentrated essential oils extracted from various parts of different plants are used for their therapeutic properties. Essential oils can be administered via the skin in massage, in the bath or in a compress, via the mucous membranes in a douche or pessary, and via the respiratory tract through inhalation. Gastrointestinal administration is advocated in some cases, although this is generally only used by experienced clinical aromatherapists.

Although aromatherapy in the UK was originally seen as part of the beauty therapy business, it is now an established element of the complementary medicine field and was identified as one of the supportive therapies within the 'top ten' therapies recognized by the British Medical Association (1993) and the Foundation for Integrated Medicine (1997). Essential oils and herbal medicines have become highly successful commercial enterprises and clinical aromatherapy is increasingly being integrated into conventional health care.

Within maternity care pregnant women frequently request information and advice regarding the safe and appropriate use of essential oils. Indeed, the incorporation of complementary therapies into midwifery practice is estimated to be as high as 34% (NHS Confederation 1997), with by far the largest proportion being aromatherapy, often combined with massage and reflexology.

Complementary therapies in general and aromatherapy in particular offer women more choices for coping with the physiological symptoms of pregnancy and the postnatal period and for easing pain and discomfort in labour, and affords them greater control over their own health care, in keeping with the philosophy of the *Changing Childbirth* report (Department of Health 1993). Evaluation and audit of maternity care is encouraging midwives to question the necessity of many traditional practices and to adapt care accordingly, facilitating a return to the nurturing aspect of being 'with woman'.

Aromatherapy as a profession has made great strides in recent years and the issues of education, regulation, research and integration are being addressed in line with the recommendations of the report published by the Foundation for Integrated Medicine (1997). Generically trained aromatherapists are choosing to specialize in particular client groups and undergoing the additional training required to enable them to practise safely and appropriately.

Historical perspectives

It is known that plants and their essences have been used for thousands of years, both for perfumes and for their therapeutic properties. The term 'aromatherapie' was not used until the early twentieth century when Gattefosse began his experiments into the medicinal uses of essential oils, after burning his hand and discovering that lavender oil acted as an analgesic, antibacterial and wound-healing agent.

In ancient Egypt, embalming and mummification of the dead was achieved with essential oils, which were found to preserve, disinfect and deodorize the bodies. Cleopatra is thought to have seduced Mark Anthony with her lavish use of perfumes. The ancient Greeks also applied aromatic oils to their bodies as perfumes and medicines and spread them around places of worship as incense. Medicinal use of plants in India dates back over 5000 years and is still the basis of Ayurvedic medicine. There are many accounts of Roman centurions benefiting from the therapeutic properties of plants, for example chewing fennel seeds to suppress hunger as they marched to battle. The Bible also has several references to aromatic oils that were used to anoint or massage the feet – Mary Magdalen anointed Jesus with spikenard ointment before the Last Supper.

Knowledge gained from the Egyptians and Indians by the Greeks, especially around the time of Hippocrates over 400 years BC, was recorded as a means of passing information to future generations. In around AD 100 the Roman, Dioscorides, compiled a 'materia medica' with details of several hundred plants. During the same period the Persian, Ibn Sina, known to us as Avicenna, is credited with discovering the method of distillation of essential oils and contributing several authoritative texts on their properties. In the Middle Ages European influences strengthened, with herbs and spices helping to ward off the Black Death in the fourteenth century. Further developments in phytotherapy (plant therapy) and perfumery occurred in the sixteenth century in Switzerland, France, Germany and Italy, and in the seventeenth century in Britain when Culpepper wrote his famous *Herbal*.

Unfortunately several factors contributed to the decline in the use of plants in the eighteenth century. Industrialization led to greater urbanization where people had little access to land for cultivating herbs. The chemical and pharmaceutical sciences were also developing, although ironically the very drugs that were eventually manufactured synthetically originated from plant substances – and there is now a return to searching out new drugs that can be manufactured from plants. Medicine, too, had become a male-dominated profession and in obstetrics the status of the midwife was at an all-time low. Plants that had previously been harvested and administered by midwives and other women who had worked as healers were now viewed with scorn and scepticism by doctors and dismissed as witchcraft.

The decline continued into the early twentieth century. During the Second World War the acreage available for growing plants was much reduced, especially in Germany, Austria and Hungary, although at the same time Valnet, considered to be the 'father' of modern aromatherapy, used essential oils to treat wounded soldiers in France. However, during the late twentieth century phytotherapy re-emerged both as herbal medicine and as aromatherapy.

This renaissance of the therapeutic uses of plants appears to be in response to a number of factors. First, it must be acknowledged that ortho-dox medicine does not have all the answers – certain carcinomas and new viral infections such as human immunodeficiency virus (HIV) and myalgic encephalitis continue to defy medical science. Second, the dislike of the side-effects of pharmaceutical preparations is causing people to look for alternatives to drugs, especially during pregnancy when many drugs are contraindicated. Third, healthcare consumers are far more willing to chal-lenge the decisions of their doctors and no longer merely to accept the views of the experts. Fourth, patients and clients want to be more involved in their own care; they want to work in partnership with professionals in order to retain more control over their health and wellbeing. Nowhere is this more apparent than in maternity care, where service users are gener-ally fit, healthy, young women. The change in the roles of women in the late twentieth century has much to do with this new assertiveness, espe-cially as greater numbers of women pursue careers, in which they may achieve a high level of seniority and power, before pausing, often in their late twenties or thirties, to have a family. Added to this is a dissatisfaction with the overburdened National Health Service (NHS) which has led to a trend towards the use of self-help strategies. While many people may opt to consult complementary practitioners with specialist expertise such as acupuncture or osteopathy, herbal, homeopathic and aromatherapy reme-dies are most readily accessible and are deemed, somewhat inaccurately, to be safer than other therapies.

Science and art Aromatherapy has now developed into a profession encompassing many different elements ranging from the purely scientific to the truly artistic. An understanding of the biological sciences of chemistry, pharmacology, and anatomy and physiology with related pathology, is vital to the safe use of essential oils within clinical aromatherapy. The artistic elements of aro-matherapy include the aesthetic blending of essential oils, competence in their methods of administration, especially full body massage, and perhaps an understanding of the principles of energies with which essential oils are thought to be imbued. Aromatology is a form of aromatic medicine that focuses on natural plant substances to treat a variety of conditions, but which does not rely on their administration by full body massage; the use of essential oils for pregnant, labouring and newly delivered mothers and their babies is perhaps closer to aromatology than aromatherapy. Essential oils can offer an extremely beneficial and enjoyable means of treating the many physiological discomforts of pregnancy and early parenthood and for dealing with discomfort in labour.

However, it is important not to forget the overall philosophy of aromatherapy: as with all complementary therapies, it is the interrelationship between the body, mind and spirit that makes aromatherapy an holistic therapy. It is possible to view essential oils simply as another form of pharmacological agent with which to treat physiological symptoms and pathological conditions, but while there is much recently available research on their metabolism and excretion, together with evidence of their claimed therapeutic qualities, there is also an increasing amount of investigation into the psychological effects of the oils.

The Foundation for Integrated Medicine's report (1997) focused on four areas for debate regarding the greater integration of complementary therapies into conventional health care: education and training; regulation; research; and delivery of services. These can be discussed in relation to clinical aromatherapy for pregnancy and childbirth.

Education and training

Maternity-related aromatherapy should involve an in-depth study of *both* clinical specialities, and any professional caring for these women and their babies must have a thorough understanding of all aspects of care – a knowledge of anatomical and physiological changes and potential pathological conditions that may occur, together with an appreciation of the conventional maternity care system that the mothers will be accessing (see Box 1.1). This must be combined with a comprehensive knowledge of both the science and the art of aromatherapy so that an appropriate application of conventional with complementary medicine can be made to ensure safe use of essential oils. The extent to which an individual practitioner needs to study each aspect will be dependent on their professional background; for example midwives will already have an understanding of pregnancy-related anatomy and physiology and of the maternity services, whereas aromatherapists should have a working knowledge of how, why and where essential oils work.

It is not acceptable for midwives to add 'aromatherapy' to their repertoire of skills in order to extend their practice without acknowledging the specific implications of using the oils in pregnancy; nor should general practitioners or obstetricians mistakenly assume that the oils are merely relaxants with which to pamper women and therefore disregard maternal enquiries regarding their use. Similarly aromatherapists must not presume

---

Box 1.1 Requisite components of maternity-related aromatherapy education and training

Maternity-related
◆ Anatomy and physiology of pregnancy, labour and puerperium

◆ Health promotion principles and concepts of health

◆ Psychology of childbirth and basic counselling skills

◆ Understanding of research methodologies and application of research findings

◆ Appreciation of healthcare ethics, legal aspects and professional accountability

◆ Knowledge of contemporary antenatal, intrapartum and postnatal care

◆ Understanding of role parameters of all professionals involved in maternity care

Aromatherapy-related
◆ Philosophy of complementary medicine

◆ Anatomy and physiology of skin, sense of touch, olfaction, respiration

◆ Related pharmacology and pharmacokinetics

◆ Basic chemical concepts and specific chemistry of essential and base oils

◆ Therapeutic properties of essential oils and related research

◆ Methods of administration

◆ Methods of blending

---

that a generic qualification equips them automatically to specialize in treating pregnant and newly delivered women and their babies, without an understanding of the limitations of their therapy and their role and an up-to-date knowledge of maternity care and the relevant biological sciences.

The Aromatherapy Organisations Council (see Regulation, below) has defined a core curriculum for aromatherapy training covering 180 classroom hours, comprising 80 h of aromatherapy, 60 h of massage and 40 h of anatomy and physiology. A minimum of 10–15 case studies must be completed, involving at least 50 hours of treatment, collated over a period of no less than 9 months. Managers of NHS maternity services who may be exploring the possibility of providing aromatherapy for women, either by midwives achieving additional qualifications or by contracting with external aromatherapists, should be guided not by the end certificate (and letters after a name), but by the educational process through which the person has been.

Regulation Until recently, education of aromatherapists has been something of a minefield with so many schools offering such a variety of qualifications that it has been impossible to identify those of best quality. This situation has changed in the last few years in response to an acknowledgement that a system of national regulation is required. Most schools of aromatherapy belong to one of a small number of registering bodies. All of these have corporate membership of the Aromatherapy Organisations Council (AOC), which represents the interests of both the public and around 5000 aromatherapists (Baker 1997). Although it is still not mandatory for aromatherapists to be registered with member institutions of the AOC, registration provides a recognizable regulatory mechanism that facilitates selection of good quality courses, reputable practitioners and suitable qualifications. The aims of the AOC include unification of the aromatherapy profession and training standards, as well as provision of a collective voice to negotiate with government and other professional organizations. The AOC also serves as a public watchdog and offers mediation and arbitration for disputes involving aromatherapy organisations, as well as initiating, supporting or sponsoring research into aromatherapy (Baker 1997).

Therapists affiliated to the AOC are required to work within a Code of Ethics and Practice similar to the Codes of Conduct for statutorily recognized health professionals such as midwives, nurses, doctors and physiotherapists. Failure to comply could lead to disciplinary action and exclusion from the AOC. Although under current law the individual could continue to practise as an aromatherapist, he or she would be unable to obtain personal professional indemnity insurance and therefore should not be contracted to provide therapy within mainstream services.

It is not compulsory for midwives wishing to incorporate the use of a limited number of essential oils into their practice to be fully qualified aromatherapists. *The Scope of Professional Practice* document (UK Central Council 1992a) facilitates, rather than restricts, the acquisition of new skills so long as they are in the best interests of patients and clients, are in response to their needs and do not fragment or compromise existing aspects of professional care. Midwives are personally accountable for their practice, must recognize the boundaries within which they work, including their own limitations, and must be able to justify their actions. The *Midwives' Rules and Code of Practice* (UK Central Council 1998) acknowledges that certain new skills may become integral to the roles of all midwives while others are developed as part of the specialist role of some midwives. The Code emphasizes the need for sound contemporary knowledge, client consent and the right of clients to self-administer substances such as essential oils or to refer to a complementary practitioner. Midwives who are unsure about the effect of a particular oil or its potential interaction with drugs should contact the relevant expert practitioner. Midwives who wish to use essential oils in their practice must be able to demonstrate that their knowledge and skills are as good as the scientific evidence currently available. Essential oils should be treated with the same respect given to drugs and midwives must abide by the standards laid down for the administration of medicines (UK Central Council 1992b). Midwives planning to utilize a limited number of essential oils for specifically defined purposes, who have the permission of their employing authority to do so and are therefore covered by vicarious liability (see below), will usually be covered also by the personal professional indemnity insurance of their professional organization or trades union.

Those midwives who are also aromatherapists may only use essential oils as part of their midwifery care if they have permission of their employing authority. Failure to do so will, in the event of a claim for negligence being brought, invalidate the individual's personal professional indemnity insurance and the trust's vicarious liability. The midwife who chooses to practise aromatherapy independently must differentiate the two roles; if he or she is consulted as an aromatherapist by a pregnant woman then the midwife must provide *aromatherapy* care only unless he or she has also notified the intention to practise as a midwife in an independent capacity. Additionally if a midwife wishes to advertise aromatherapy services then he or she should not rely on his or her midwifery qualification to enhance credibility and respectability of the aromatherapy qualification (UK Central Council 1996). It must also be understood that aromatherapy or other complementary therapy qualifications *cannot* be added to an individual's entry on the statutory register and that the UK Central Council for Nursing, Midwifery and Health Visiting has no jurisdiction over what constitutes an acceptable course for a profession that they do not regulate.

Research

Evidence-based practice is vital to the provision of safe effective health care. It is true to say that some aspects of conventional medicine remain largely unevaluated, with the exception of pharmaceutical substances, a system that came into being following the thalidomide disaster in the 1960s. However, orthodox practitioners are traditionally more in tune with the notion of statistically significant evidence to support practice, whereas it has only been in the past few years that good quality research into aromatherapy has begun, especially clinical trials.

One of the problems for aromatherapy, as for other complementary therapies, is to demonstrate not only whether the essential oils are effective, but also how they work and whether they are safe. The biomedical sciences have long depended on randomized controlled double-blind trials and view these as the 'gold standard' by which all clinical research should be measured. However, many complementary therapies cannot be investigated in this way because the very nature of their effectiveness is based on factors that cannot be double-blinded, for example the use of touch. Much research is being undertaken into the effectiveness of aromatherapy in an attempt to determine whether it works because of the essential oil constituents, the method of administration, especially massage, or the therapeutic relationship between client and therapist. There is greater reliance within complementary medicine on collective and collaborative case reporting as a means of demonstrating effectiveness – and apparent safety – of essential oils. Unfortunately it would seem that, despite reservations about conventional medical practice being based totally on evidence, complementary medicine has to prove itself twice over in order to be considered valid, effective and safe.

In maternity care there has been little research involving the administration of essential oils and that which has been undertaken has been based on the premise that any oils used in pregnancy or labour are generally considered to be safe because there is no documented evidence to the contrary. Trials on the potential teratogenic or abortifacient effects of essential oils have been carried out only on animals and the huge ethical problems of researching the administration of essential oils on pregnant women means that there is a dearth of knowledge on the subject. Pharmaceutical companies spend many years and a great deal of money on researching new drugs to demonstrate beyond doubt that their products are safe for the public, and there are occasions when the potential side-effects on humans are found to be so unacceptable as to warrant the discontinuation of a drug's development. The costs of this system, if applied to aromatherapy, would be prohibitive and, in any case, the proportion of essential oil destined for clinical aromatherapy is only about 10% of the total oil production (the bulk being used in the perfumery and food industries). It is not possible to patent natural products so there is no incentive for individual companies to undertake the research with its accompanying expense, and if they chose to do so, essential oils currently available would have to be withdrawn from sale until proven to be acceptable.

Delivery of services

Expectant mothers may come into contact with aromatherapy via a variety of routes. They may already have used essential oils or may have consulted an aromatherapist prior to becoming pregnant; they may have learned recently of the potential value of aromatherapy in pregnancy and wish to self-administer essential oils or seek help from a professional aromatherapist; or they may be offered essential oils by practitioners of orthodox maternity care, primarily midwives. It is therefore necessary to consider these different scenarios in the light of ensuring safe and appropriate maternity *and* aromatherapy care for women.

Each healthcare professional with whom the mother comes into contact has a vital but different role to play in her care. Legally the only persons who should provide antenatal, labour and postnatal care, except in an emergency, are midwives or doctors, or those in training, under supervision.

The *Changing Childbirth* report (Department of Health 1993) investigated the state of maternity care in the UK and made recommendations for improvements that would ensure greater choice for women with consequently more control over their own health and improve continuity of care and communication between healthcare professionals and mothers. The report recommended that women should have a designated 'lead professional' responsible for their overall wellbeing; this is most frequently the midwife, but may, if the mother chooses or her condition warrants it, be her general practitioner or the consultant obstetrician.

Midwives   Midwives are independently accountable practitioners who may or may not also be qualified nurses. They are experts in the care of women with uncomplicated pregnancies, normal labours and puerperia and will generally care for the mother and baby from conception to 4–6 weeks after the birth. The majority of midwives are employed by the National Health Service and may work in either hospital maternity departments, community practice or a combination of both. Many midwives now work in teams or caseloads, offering women exposure to a limited number of midwives whom they can come to know during pregnancy in preparation for the birth. A few midwives work in private practice and contract directly with women who choose to pay for the services of one or two designated midwives. In the UK about 70% of deliveries are conducted by midwives who will be the most senior professionals present. All midwives are bound by statutory guidelines and must adhere to the *Midwives' Rules and Code of Practice* (UK Central Council 1998) and other regulations.

Midwives are in an ideal position to incorporate essential oils into the care of childbearing women, but this must be balanced against other priorities of care, especially with the constraints of time and staffing levels. They may be qualified in aromatherapy or entitled to use a limited number of oils, or may be caring for women wishing to self-administer essential oils. The principal benefit to mothers in the care of midwives using or advising on aromatherapy is the element of continuity of care, rather than the fragmentation that may arise if other professionals (i.e. independent aromatherapists) are involved in their care. However, while this may be particularly pertinent at the time of labour and delivery, it is unlikely that many midwives will be in a position to offer regular antenatal and postnatal aromatherapy, especially that administered through full body massage.

The accountability of the midwife in relation to the use of aromatherapy has already been highlighted. Midwifery managers should consider the necessity of developing locally relevant protocols to safeguard both the health of women in their care and the professional integrity of midwifery staff using aromatherapy. Box 1.2 lists possible inclusions in such a protocol.

Although consultant obstetricians are unlikely to be in a position to sign 'standing orders' unless they are qualified aromatherapists, it may be pertinent for midwives to discuss with their medical colleagues the use of aromatherapy within the maternity unit and to make them aware of protocols for aromatherapy in midwifery. It is *not*, however, necessary for midwives to obtain 'permission' from consultant obstetricians to use aromatherapy in ways that fall within the boundaries of their own midwifery practice.

General practitioners   General practitioners (GPs) are community-based doctors with a defined local caseload, who usually care for the whole family, attending to their everyday health needs. They specialize in differentiating minor from major health conditions and will, when necessary, refer patients for more specialist care. Many GPs are qualified in obstetrics and gynaecology and are able to offer antenatal care to women within their practice, although they must refer any women with complications to

---

Box 1.2   Points to be considered in drawing up a protocol

Training The type of aromatherapy training that is locally acceptable may need to be specified (see Education and training, above).

Staff It may be appropriate to maintain a 'live' register of midwives entitled to use aromatherapy in their practice, whether they are fully qualified aromatherapists or adequately prepared to administer specified oils.

Oils Managers may wish to specify a limited number of essential and base oils that can be used for the client group, which will facilitate monitoring of costs, effects and any possible side-effects. The number of oils to be used in a blend may also be defined since, although combining oils promotes synergistic action (see Chapter 6), it is more difficult to identify causative oils in the event of adverse reactions.

Dosage This would include the permitted doses of blends and the amount any one mother may receive in one day. Bottles should be clearly labelled with doses.

Route of administration This may alter according to the symptom being treated, for instance constipation may be treated with abdominal massage of essential oils while perineal trauma would respond better to the addition of essential oils to the bath or bidet. Health and safety regulations may prohibit certain methods of administration such as vaporization using candles.

Client selection Categories of women who may or may not be treated with essential oils should be identified. 'High-risk' mothers may be excluded from aromatherapy treatment, although what constitutes 'high risk' should be determined locally.

Conditions It may be advisable to restrict to physiological symptoms those conditions that can be treated with essential oils, in keeping with the normal parameters of the midwife's role.

Restrictions Any locally agreed restrictions should be documented.

Blending Staff responsible for blending essential and base oils should be identified by name, as well as the amount and frequency of blending.

Storage Designated areas for storing oils should be allocated, in accordance with health and safety measures.

Approved documentation It will need to be decided whether client consent is to be recorded in writing or can be accepted verbally. Records of the essential and base oils administered should be maintained either in the normal midwifery notes or the main hospital notes if these are different or on a separate form.

---

a consultant obstetrician. In reality the roles of the midwife and the general practitioner partially overlap, but some women like to maintain contact with their GPs, particularly if they already know them well.

Some general practitioners contract the services of aromatherapists on a sessional basis, but care should be taken with regards to the qualifications and relevant experience of individual therapists. GPs should also consider issues such as the room to be used for aromatherapy, which should be well ventilated, with a lockable cupboard for the storage of oils in keeping with regulations on the Control of Substances Hazardous to Health (COSHH) (see Health and safety, Chapter 5). It is desirable that the room is not required immediately after use by the aromatherapist to avoid inhalation of lingering essential oil vapours by other patients. GPs should also consider whether they are *referring* women for aromatherapy or *delegating* to the therapist one aspect of care that they have prescribed.

Obstetricians   Obstetricians are doctors who have specialized in women's health and usually combine maternity care with gynaecology. Hospital teams of obstetricians are headed by consultants with senior and junior registrars training to specialize in this field. There may also be senior house officers who, while not newly qualified doctors, will be novices in the area of obstetrics and will be undergoing training with their more senior medical colleagues and with midwives. Some of these house officers may intend to specialize in obstetrics or may be training to become general practitioners.

The most fundamental difference between midwives and obstetricians is that midwives are the experts in *normal midwifery* while doctors are experts in *abnormal obstetrics*. There is some blurring of the boundaries between their roles that may differ according to where they work, but generally women will only see an obstetrician if and when problems occur.

Obstetricians should be aware that expectant women use aromatherapy and appreciate that they cannot afford to be complacent, antagonistic or confrontational about this or other complementary therapies. Anticipation of demand for information about and treatment with essential oils, even in areas where there has hitherto been little, should prompt active, constructive, multidisciplinary discussion on the issues of concern for the maternity care team. Obstetricians must acknowledge the limitations of their own knowledge and be prepared to consult experts in aromatherapy on this subject. However, they may wish to be involved in defining any restrictions in the use of essential oils within a maternity department (see Box 1.2 above).

As more women become interested and involved in aromatherapy it may become necessary for midwives, general practitioners or obstetricians to ask routine questions at the first antenatal appointment about whether a mother is using any essential oils. This could quite easily be included in the questions on medication. A policy of openness about clients' use of complementary therapies will facilitate communication between mothers and their carers before a potentially dangerous situation develops.

Clinical aromatherapists   Clinical aromatherapists have undertaken training in the therapeutic administration of essential oils, including the relevant science and art of their profession. Most aromatherapy courses provide a good basic coverage of the anatomy of the whole body and some of the related physiology (see Education and training, above). Post-qualification courses and study days are available on specialist elements of aromatherapy practice and it would be wise for any therapist intending to specialize in the care of pregnant women to study the subject in depth.

All aromatherapists should be registered with one of the regulatory bodies, most of which are corporate members of the Aromatherapy Organisations Council. Any therapist attempting to contract with an NHS maternity service, or any midwifery manager exploring the feasibility of employing an aromatherapist on a sessional basis, must ensure that the therapist is covered by personal professional indemnity insurance.

Aromatherapists who practise independently and who may be consulted by women who are pregnant should attempt to develop good communication links with local maternity service providers. Their pregnant clients should be encouraged to inform their midwives or doctors that they are receiving aromatherapy and the therapist would be wise to write to the general practitioner, midwife or obstetrician to clarify what treatment is being given. While all professionals are part of a team, collaborative working can only be achieved by good communication and an acknowledgement by each professional of his or her role within the team and the limitations of that role.

Aromatherapists *must* appreciate that legally the midwife or doctor is primarily responsible for the care of the expectant or new mother and her baby. There may be occasions when, despite the views of the aromatherapist that essential oils could be beneficial, it is inappropriate to insist on their use. An example of potential conflict would be when the mother is experiencing inadequate uterine contractions in labour that the aromatherapist feels could be stimulated by using essential oils, but which have resulted from uterine inertia due to an obstructed labour. It would indeed be dangerous to attempt to accelerate contractions if the size or position of the fetus indicated the impossibility of a vaginal delivery – excessive uterine action could cause it to rupture, leading to death of the baby and possibly the mother. Any essential oils administered by the aromatherapist, especially during the acute episode of labour and delivery, must be with the knowledge and consent not only of the mother but also of the midwife or doctor.

Some maternity units will have specific policies about the involvement of therapists from outside the NHS system, which identify the role boundaries of each professional and require evidence of both qualification and the possession of indemnity insurance cover. Aromatherapists accompanying women into the labour ward may be asked to sign a form to this effect acknowledging their understanding that the trust's vicarious liability cannot apply to any claims resulting from negligence on the part of the therapist.

Mothers   Mothers are the very focus of the maternity services: without pregnant and childbearing women there would, of course, be no service. Women have a right to administer to themselves substances such as essential oils, but may need professional assistance to use them safely. Midwives, general practitioners and obstetricians should facilitate the empowerment of women in all aspects of maternity care, not only related to the use of aromatherapy. A policy of openness among professionals will prevent mothers from feeling the need to use essential oils clandestinely, perhaps with the risk of interactions with drugs or exacerbation of complications. Women should be made aware of the safe uses of essential oils during pregnancy, labour and the puerperium and for their newborn babies and should feel able to ask questions without fear of scepticism, dismissal or disparagement. However, mothers must also acknowledge their own responsibilities for their health and that of their babies, and be guided by the experts. If a woman is considering using essential oils during pregnancy and labour but is being cared for by midwives unfamiliar with aromatherapy, the midwives cannot be accountable for her self-administration. Midwives should document that the mother is intending to use essential oils and record that she is doing so on her own responsibility, until such time as expert aromatherapy advice has been sought, in accordance with the professional obligations of midwives (UK Central Council 1998).

Conclusion Aromatherapy offers a wonderful means of helping women to cope with the physiological symptoms of pregnancy and early parenthood and to ease discomfort and pain in labour. It is a gentle therapy that fosters a sense of nurturing and a return to the very essence of childbirth as a normal but significant life event. Helping women to enjoy the benefits of essential oils gives them a sense of empowerment and achievement that enables them to reflect on their childbearing periods with satisfaction.

Aromatherapy can be incorporated into conventional maternity care by midwives, who may either administer the oils themselves or assist women who wish to self-administer to do so safely and effectively. General practitioners and obstetricians are also in a position to direct women to sources of accurate information regarding safe usage. Independent aromatherapists may increasingly be involved in caring for pregnant, labouring and newly delivered mothers and can, by developing good communication with orthodox practitioners, establish links to ensure that all women have the opportunity to experience the positive effects of essential oils. Only by continuing to strengthen this partnership between conventional and complementary care, and so providing the best from both systems, can mothers be assured of the highest standards of maternity care.

Chapter 2

Extraction, Quality and Storage of Essential Oils

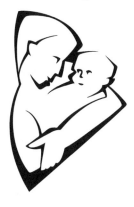

Extraction of essential oils from plants

Essential oils are the highly volatile fluid constituents in plants, usually found in tiny droplets in the veins, glands, glandular hairs and sacs. Their function in the plant is to act as regulators, hormones and catalysts, and to assist the plant in adapting to environments that would normally be stressful, with a consequent increase in growth. Essential oils also act as a protection for the plant against diseases, parasites and, in very hot areas, the sun. Some essential oils help to attract insects for pollination and may work as natural weedkillers on the surrounding soil. They are often coloured, do not dissolve in water but mix well in vegetable oils, fats and waxes, and fairly well in alcohol.

Some plants yield a minute amount of essential oil compared with others; for example, over 100 kg of rose petals are required to produce just 50–80 g of the essential oil, which makes true rose oil extremely expensive. The chemical constituents of an individual type of essential oil can vary according to the geographical terrain and climate, the time of day and the season. An investigation into *Rosmarinus officinalis* (rosemary) demonstrated similarity of chemical components in oils obtained from Hungary and Germany, but there was an absence of camphor and borneol in the sample from England (Hethelyi et al 1987). An exploration of ten samples of rosemary from British oil producers also demonstrated considerable differences in chemical constituents and showed that rosemary was often adulterated by the addition of eucalyptus and camphor oils (Svoboda & Deans 1990) in an attempt to replace the constituents that were missing.

Different parts of plants will produce different essential oils; for instance, from the orange tree can be extracted essential oils of orange (from the rind), neroli (from the orange blossom) and petitgrain (from the twigs). Many of the essential oils derived from culinary herbs, such as sage, rosemary and marjoram, have been extracted from the leaves. Others are extracted from the fruit, especially the citrus oils, from the flowers (neroli, camomile), seeds (carrot seed, black pepper) or the bark or inner part of a tree (sandalwood, rosewood).

The method of extraction will depend on the part of the plant from which the essential oil is derived and the difficulty in so doing. Extraction of citrus essences is a relatively simple process of expression and many readers will themselves have been able to extract the essence from an orange, merely in the act of peeling the fruit: the spurt of liquid is essence from the peel, not juice from the flesh of the orange. Most essential oils are extracted through a process of steam distillation but the opposite extreme is the complicated solvent extraction process for oils from delicate petals such as jasmine, neroli or rose, for they would be damaged both by expression or steam distillation.

Steam distillation The original process of distillation is attributed to the Arab physician Avicenna, although it is possible that the ancient Egyptians used a similar process. In principle, the procedure has changed little since its origins.

Using a specially constructed still, boiled water is turned to steam which then softens the plant tissues allowing the essential oils to escape. The essential oil vaporizes and rises to pass into the vapour pipe, where it is cooled and a mixture of oil and water is collected. This can be separated fairly easily by means of a filter system or centrifugal separator (Fig. 2.1).

The actual process of distillation is simple, although some plants have to undergo the process several times in order to obtain the full yield of essential oil. The oil producer needs skill and experience to ensure that the plants are prepared appropriately to obtain optimum yields. In some plants, such as sandalwood and cedarwood, the essential oil-containing cells are situated deep within hard tissue so that the chips of wood have to be almost powdered down to rupture the cell walls for the essential oil to be accessed. This is known as comminution.

Fig. 2.1. *Simple steam distillation apparatus.*

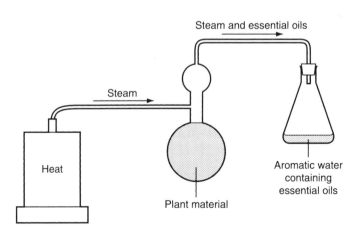

Timing of the extraction process is important too, as some plants need immediate distillation to avoid the essential oil being lost or destroyed, e.g. melissa. Some plants may be left to remove excess water before distillation, e.g. lavender, and others may be completely dried out, e.g. black pepper seeds. However, Watt (personal communication, 1996) believes that steam distillation, with its accompanying heat, can destroy many of the chemicals in the essential oils, thereby affecting their therapeutic properties. He advocates the use of cold processing to extract the best quality essential oils.

A method of extraction which works on a principle similar to that of a coffee percolator, called hydrodiffusion, is being used in France and appears to produce more aromatic and highly coloured essential oils than those produced by steam distillation.

Carbon dioxide extraction An extremely expensive method of using compressed carbon dioxide as a solvent to extract the essential oils has also been available since the early 1980s, producing oils closer to those in the actual plant. Although the equipment costs several million pounds it has been used in a few units in France, Japan, Germany and America, and could be used commercially in the near future. This method has the advantage of using a lower temperature so that the essential oils are not damaged by heat, and it is much quicker than steam distillation, which can take up to 48 h to complete, with the risk of some oxidation of the essential oils.

Cold expression This process is used to extract oils from citrus fruits, although lime oil is more often distilled than expressed.

Crushing of the whole fruit followed by separation of the essential oil from the juice and peel is one method of expression. Alternatively the outer rind of the fruit may be abraded and the essence collected after centrifugal separation from the debris, a method used to obtain bergamot oil.

Expressed oils usually have a small amount of antioxidant added to them to prevent rapid deterioration, but the storage life of these oils is still fairly short, about 3 months. The essences should be stored in a cool dark place, preferably in the refrigerator, as light and heat will initiate the degeneration process.

Solvent extraction The original method of extraction used for delicate flowers such as roses, jasmine or orange blossom is called enfleurage. It involved pressing the petals between layers of fat until the fat was saturated with essential oils that were then removed by distillation.

In plants where heat or water may cause damage to the essential oils, solvent extraction is now used to produce essential oils classed as absolutes or resinoids, which are highly concentrated aromatic materials. Resins are the exudates from trees that partially or totally solidify on mixing with air. Solvents such as hydrocarbons are used to extract the aromatic material from the resin; these are later filtered off and removed by distillation.

Some authorities believe that absolutes are not suitable for use in aromatherapy and should be used only in perfumery as they almost always retain some of the solvent (Lavabre 1990, p. 19), although this should be under ten parts per thousand (Ryman 1991, p. 10). Others suggest that they may be used for therapeutic work but that practitioners should be aware of the possible sensitivity caused by the solvent residue that may occur in some people (Price 1993, p. 21).

Occasionally solvent extraction is preferred over steam distillation in order to produce an absolute with a different type of aroma from the essential oil. For example, the perfumery industry may use an absolute of lavender for a variety of purposes, rather than the essential oil. When an absolute is used in aromatherapy it is vital to purchase from a reputable supplier who can account for its origins, for the extra cost involved in production can lead some producers to adulterate the absolute with a cheaper essential oil or a synthetic substitute.

Quality of essential oils

It is imperative when using essential oils therapeutically that they are of the highest possible quality. This is a problem, however, as the essential oil producers supply the vast majority of their oils to the perfumery and food industries with only a small proportion of business going to the aromatherapy market. Although there are obviously stringent quality controls for these other industries, they do not have the same priorities and it would be an extremely costly exercise for producers to adapt equipment and procedures for such analyses as are required by aromatherapists.

It has already been mentioned that the chemical profile of an essential oil can be affected by a variety of factors such as climate. The addition of chemical fertilizers and weedkillers can also, of course, adversely affect the plant and thus the essential oil. Perhaps the only sure way to obtain the best quality oil is to find a supplier of organic essential oils, although Watt (personal communication, 1996) disputes this, stating that there is little evidence that so-called organically grown plants produce essential oils that have significantly different (i.e. more effective) properties. It is true that 'you get what you pay for' in aromatherapy, but this is surely in the interests of clients receiving the oils.

It is useful here to compare essential oils to pharmacological drugs. Pharmaceutical companies apply for patents for drugs in which the active ingredients are blended to a specific 'secret' – and later, patented – recipe. Similar drugs are available in a generic form but the exact combination of chemical ingredients will differ slightly and may affect an individual differently. An example of this can be seen in the varying responses one person may have to two different brands of iron tablet.

In aromatherapy an individual essential oil is selected for its known therapeutic properties, due to the balance of chemical components. If a particular batch of essential oil lacks some of those chemicals, perhaps due to climatic conditions (essential oils are like wine, there are good years and bad years), some producers may attempt to add the missing ingredient, either from another essential oil or with a synthetic substance. It is also known that certain of the more expensive oils or absolutes are adulterated with cheaper oils that have a similar odour. For instance, rose may have rose geranium, palmarosa, lemongrass or even synthetic chemicals such as stearine or a terpenic alcohol added in an attempt to raise profits.

An increasing number of essential oil suppliers now provide a written analysis of the actual oil being sold with a guarantee of quality control mechanisms. When essential oils are as pure as can be found, the therapist will in fact need to use less to achieve the same results – a little like some of the advertisments for washing-up liquid seen on television. Organic or biological essential oils are issued with a certificate of proof, although it must be recognized that, despite organic growing methods without the use of pesticides, it is still possible for the plants to have been exposed to environmental contamination outside the control of the grower, such as the Chernobyl disaster.

Analysis of essential oils
Essential oils can be analysed using a system called gas chromatography. The original process was invented in the 1920s to separate chlorophylls from plants but was not really developed further until the 1960s; by the 1980s the process had become much more sophisticated.

Chromatography in its simplest form involves the application of a thin layer of silica gel to a glass plate, to which is added, near one end of the plate, a minute amount of the substance to be analysed. The glass plate is inserted into a lidded receptacle containing a solvent that rises by capillary action up the plate. As the solvent moves up the plate, the solute (in this case, essential oils) is washed up the plate with it. The analysis depends on the fact that different solutes move upwards at different rates, thus a 'fingerprint' of an essential oil can be made. Technological advances now mean that chromatography can be performed using computerized machinery (Fig. 2.2).

Gas chromatography is similar in principle to the simple chromatography described above but uses gases instead of silica-coated plates. A modern development is the use of high-performance liquid chromatography, which may replace gas chromatography in the foreseeable future.

Chromatographic analysis is undertaken when the purity of an essential oil is in question. The analysis of the oil is matched against the known profile of the named oil, and may show the presence of undesirable constituents.

A case is known to this author of a nurse who bought some 'neroli oil' from a popular high street retailer of beauty products. After advice from a friend she added a mere three drops of the oil to her bathwater one evening. She sat in the bath for several minutes and then apparently 'blacked out' for a few seconds. She was eventually able to get out of the bath, and put her experience down to the bathwater being too hot,

Fig. 2.2. *(a)   Modern chromatography equipment.*

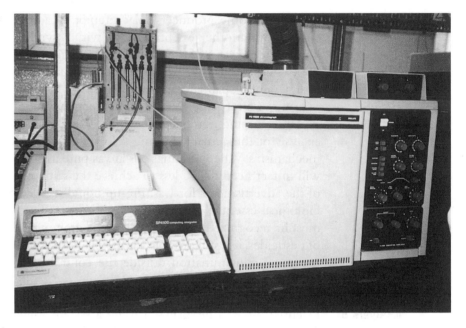

Fig. 2.2. *(b)   High-performance liquid chromatography.*

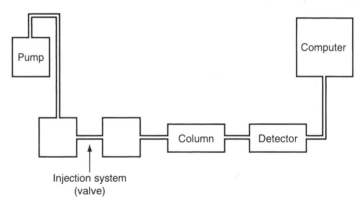

although she was accustomed to having a hot bath. A few days later she tried the oil again, using only three drops in the water as before. This time she felt herself becoming lightheaded and faint, and quickly got out of the bath.

The nurse returned the oil to the shop where she had bought it and was initially met with derision until she insisted on having the oil analysed. It was only after she left the shop that it occurred to her that she should have kept some of the oil to obtain an independent analysis. Unfortunately the report returned from the supplier did not show any contamination of the oil. However, the important fact here is that such shops do not sell essential oils; they offer a selection of aromatic oils that smell good but are not intended for therapeutic use. Although this type of shop makes no claims for the oils, it is the lack of knowledge on the part of the public that leads them to believe that aromatic oils are the same as essential oils. Furthermore, this misconception is not repudiated by the retailer and adds to the lack of credibility of aromatherapy.

Storage of essential oils

Essential oils are expensive and deserve to be kept in a way that will preserve their properties for as long as possible. They are also toxic when misused (i.e. overdosed), and from an accountability point of view should therefore be stored with the same regard to safety as drugs.

Physically, essential oils will deteriorate, or oxidize, when they are exposed to oxygen, light or changing temperatures. Essential oils are supplied in dark brown or blue bottles and should be stored in a cool dark place to avoid oxidation that can be caused by the ozone present in bright sunlight. The bottles should always be made of glass as plastic may act as a chemical catalyst and initiate degenerative changes; in addition, ultraviolet light from the sun, which could adversely affect the oils, will not penetrate through glass. Where bottles are supplied with a dropper, this should also be of glass. However, droppers with rubber tops should, for similar reasons, be stored separately from the essential oils.

It is better to purchase quantities that will be used up fairly quickly, rather than buying in bulk, which would be uneconomic if the oils are unused within their estimated therapeutic shelf-life. Most essential oils retain their properties for up to a year; after this time polymerization, the breaking up of double bonds in the compounds, may cause changes to occur, leaving a sediment (which will be a contaminant) in the base of the bottle. Some authorities consider that certain essential oils may keep for up to 2 or even 3 years if they are well stored (Lavabre 1990, p. 22), but some oils such as the citrus essences are known to have a shelf-life of only 3–6 months.

Essential oils should also be kept unblended for as long as possible because once they are mixed with a carrier oil the process of oxidation will begin. This may mean that certain of the chemicals break down to form different products, thus altering the profile of the oil and its therapeutic value. Concentrated essential oils should have the lid of the bottle firmly closed and, indeed, it is good practice, especially when carrying out a full body massage, which can take over an hour, for the blended oil to be kept covered or in a container with a lid. Water will also cause oxidation, so sprays containing essential oils should be used up within a day of mixing.

For issues related to storage of essential oils from a health and safety perspective, see Chapter 5.

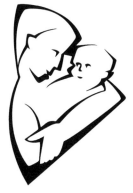

Chapter 3 **Properties and Constituents of Essential Oils**

Chemistry To appreciate the scientific nature of aromatherapy it is necessary to understand some basic chemical concepts. Chemistry is the study of matter and its properties; matter is everything that has mass and occupies space. Organic chemistry is the study of chemistry in living things, i.e. plants and animals, or perhaps it could be referred to as the study of the carbon compound, for all living things contain carbon. Inorganic chemistry refers to non-living matter and is not relevant to aromatherapy.

An *element* is a chemical substance that cannot be split into simpler substances, with all the atoms in it having the same number of protons. There are 92 natural elements, including hydrogen, carbon, nitrogen and oxygen, plus some formed by nuclear reactions. Some of these elements are gases and therefore the lightest, others are solids and two are liquids; some elements are reactive, others are not.

An *atom* is the smallest particle of an element that retains the chemical properties of that element. An atom has a nucleus containing one or more electrically positive protons and one or more neutral neutrons. Negative electrical charges (electrons) orbit around the atom, usually with two in the innermost shell and up to eight in the outermost shell of the atom. The atoms of a particular element all contain the same number of protons, and it is this unique proton number that defines the element (Fig. 3.1a).

Valency refers to the combining power of different elements as a result of the number of bonds it can make. Hydrogen can only form a single bond with another atom; therefore it is said to have a valency of 1. Oxygen has a valency of 2, so that it makes two bonds. When oxygen combines with hydrogen two hydrogen atoms are required, one for each bond. The compound formed is thus H–O–H, or H_2O, i.e. water (Fig. 3.1b).

A *compound* is formed when atoms of two or more elements are attached to each other, for example the compound carbon dioxide consists of one carbon atom and two oxygen atoms bonded together.

Fig. 3.1. *(a) Structure of an oxygen atom. There are eight protons(+ve charges) in the nucleus, which holds eight electrons (−ve charges) in orbit around it.*
(b) In the water molecule one oxygen atom combines with two hydrogen atoms. The atoms are bonded together by sharing their electrons.
(c) The charge in a water molecule is not distributed evenly − there is a small negative charge on the oxygen atom farthest from the hydrogen atoms, and small positive charges on the hydrogen atoms farthest from the oxygen atom. This results in electrostatic forces of attraction between neighbouring molecules, called hydrogen bonds (shown by dashed lines).

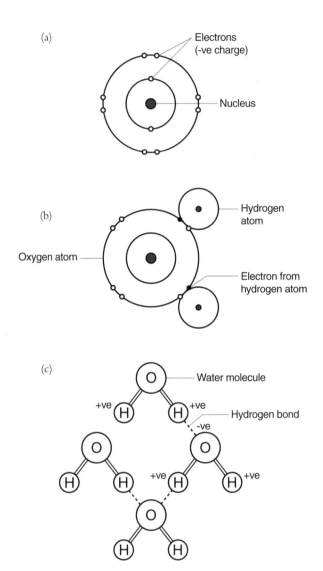

A *molecule* is the smallest part of a chemical compound that normally exists on its own and can take part in a chemical reaction. Within one compound all the molecules have the same number of atoms. The shape of a molecule affects the properties of the compound. For example, water forms a v-shaped molecule in which the electrical charge is distributed unevenly (Fig. 3.1c). This results in electrostatic forces of attraction between water molecules, which give water its high melting and boiling points relative to other molecules of a similar size.

When compounds are formed, each element must have the same number of bonds as its valency for the compound to be complete. Those molecules that are the most difficult to separate are the most stable, such as nitrogen, in which two nitrogen atoms form three bonds with each other. This differs from hydrogen molecules, in which two hydrogen atoms form a single bond with each other. The bond can easily be broken and so hydrogen molecules are unstable.

In some compounds double bonds are formed, but these are more easily broken down by chemical processes. Many of the constituents of essential oils contain double bonds, which is why factors such as light and heat cause the oils to deteriorate. Another example is the addition of essential oils to water for sprays: it is necessary to use distilled water as the presence of chlorine in tap water adversely affects the essential oils and begins the process of oxidation. Incidentally, double bonds are partly responsible for the colours of essential oils; the colour increases as the number of double bonds increases.

A *mixture* has more than one kind of molecule within it, unlike a compound which has only one type. A mixture may be separated by various processes into its individual molecules. When compounds are submitted to physical changes, such as melting, boiling or condensing, the molecules remain unchanged, but with chemical changes, for example combustion, there are large energy changes involving heat and light which result in the molecules being changed and atoms rearranged. This can be demonstrated when 1 g of magnesium is burned: due to the addition of oxygen during burning, almost 2 g of white powder are the end-product.

Volatility refers to the fact that essential oils evaporate easily and are also flammable when they come in contact with extremes of heat; this is important when considering where to store the oils. Care must also be taken when using candle burners that the essential oils do not come into direct contact with the flame.

To smell the aroma of an essential oil, at least one molecule has to evaporate and enter the nostril. Imagine, then, the number of molecules that must be present in a few drops of essential oil which evaporate in a large room, yet can be smelt by everyone present in that room. In fact 1 ml (1 cm^3) of essential oil actually contains 1×10^{22} molecules, i.e. 10 000 000 000 000 000 000 000 molecules.

Constituents of essential oils

It is the chemical constituents of essential oils that give them their therapeutic properties (Table 3.1). However, it must be remembered that a typical essential oil will contain over 100 chemical constituents, some of which may not even have been identified. Watt (personal communication, 1996) states that it is not truly possible to attribute therapeutic properties to individual chemical components, and that it is the overall combination and balance of the chemicals, coupled with the method of administration, that enables practitioners to make claims for achieving certain therapeutic benefits from the oils. When analysis of an essential oil is carried out a list of the main 'ingredients' is made; those in the largest proportions are usually placed at the beginning of the list, in the same way that lists of ingredients in food products are in percentage order.

Table 3.1
Claimed
therapeutic
properties
of some
phytochemicals

Chemical constituent	Functional group	Therapeutic property	Example of essential oil
Arbutin	Phenol	Diuretic Urinary antiseptic Antitussive	Marjoram
Benzoic acid	Phenol	Antifungal Choleretic	Benzoin
Bergapten	Coumarin	Photoxic	Bergamot
Bornyl acetate	Ester	Expectorant	Rosemary
Camphene	Monoterpene	Cholesterol-reducing	Nutmeg Cypress
Camphor	Ketone	Rubefacient Irritant Mild analgesic	Lavender Cinnamon
Carvacrol	Phenol	Antiseptic Antifungal Antihelmintic	Thyme Marjoram
Chamazulene	Sesquiterpene	Anti-inflammatory Antipyretic Antiphlogistic	Camomile
1,8-Cineole	Oxide	Expectorant Antihelmintic	Eucalyptus
Cinnamic aldehyde	Aldehyde	Lacrimatory Skin irritant	Cinnamon
Citral	Aldehyde	Antiseptic ($5 \times$ phenol)	Lemongrass
Farnesol	Alcohol	Antibacterial	Rose Camomile
Fenchone	Ketone	Counter-irritant	Fennel
Geraniol	Alcohol	Antiseptic ($7 \times$ phenol)	Geranium Rose
Limonene	Monoterpene	Sedative Expectorant Skin irritant	Lemon Orange Mandarin
Linalol	Alcohol	Antiseptic ($5 \times$ phenol)	Lavender Bergamot
Menthol	Alcohol	Mucolytic Antipruritic Carminative Analgesic	Mint oils
Zingiberene	Monoterpene	Carminative	Ginger

All essential oils are formed as the result of combinations of carbon, hydrogen and oxygen. These are the foundations of all other constituents within the oils: mono-, sesqui- and di-terpenes, alcohols, aldehydes, ketones, acids, esters, ethers, coumarins, oxides and lactones. Substances such as tannins, mucilages and flavonoids are plant constituents used therapeutically by medical herbalists but are not found in essential oils. This is partly because the extraction process usually involves the use of water, so that only small, volatile, water-insoluble substances can be isolated from the plant.

Monoterpenes   Monoterpenes are made up of two chains of five carbon atoms known as isoprenes, i.e. they contain ten atoms of carbon, together with hydrogen atoms attached to the 'arms' of the atoms; they are the smallest of the terpenoid molecules. Monoterpenes occur in almost all essential oils in varying proportions, and include camphene, limonene (Fig. 3.2), myrcene, phellandrene and pinene. As can be seen, the names all end in 'ene', making them easy to identify. They are antibacterial, especially in air, and occasionally antiviral. They are stimulating and act as a mild analgesic;

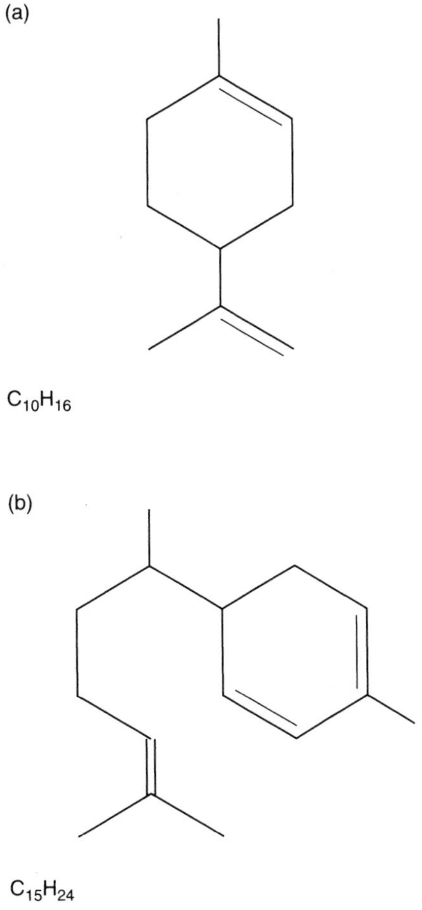

Fig. 3.2. Structure of (a) limonene and (b) zingiberene.

(a)

$C_{10}H_{16}$

(b)

$C_{15}H_{24}$

research by Lorenzetti et al (1991) found that myrcene, a constituent of lemongrass oil, appears to act as a peripheral analgesic without tolerance developing after repeated administration. Monoterpenes also have expectorant properties, as has been demonstrated by Boyd & Sheppard's (1970) investigations into camphene, a major constituent of nutmeg oil. Schafer & Schafer (1981) elicited broncholytic and secretolytic effects from an ointment containing camphene (and menthol). Monoterpenes are thought to irritate the skin in susceptible people, so should always be administered in a base oil if they are to come in contact with the skin, although Price (1993, p. 36) suggests that dextro-limonene may 'quench' the irritating effects of other constituents such as aldehyde in lemongrass oil. Monoterpenes have been found to be soluble in blood and in oil, which suggests that they will accumulate in the adipose tissues of the body. This occurs particularly when administered via the respiratory tract, as shown by Falk-Filipsson's work (1993) in which healthy men inhaled *d*-limonene in varying concentrations with a 70% respiratory uptake and a long half-life. *d*-Limonene is also thought to have potential value in detoxifying chemical carcinogens as it has been found (with geraniol, in lemongrass oil) to increase the activity of glutathione S-transferase (a detoxifying liver enzyme) in mice (Zheng et al 1993).

Sesquiterpenes   The term sesqui means 'one and a half', and sesquiterpenes contain one and a half monoterpenes, or three isoprene units of five carbon atoms. The isoprene units may be in a long chain or in a cyclical formation, such as α-farnesene found in citronella and zingiberene (Fig. 3.2) in ginger oil.

Sesquiterpenes share some similarities of action with monoterpenes, being antiseptic, antibacterial and analgesic, but they are also anti-inflammatory, antispasmodic and hypotensive, and, unlike the stimulating effects of monoterpenes, sesquiterpenes are relaxing; in addition they do not seem to be skin irritants.

Examples of sesquiterpenes include α-terpinene, β-bisabolene, farnesene and sabinene (again the names end in 'ene').

These molecules are bigger and heavier than monoterpenes and have decreased volatility; they are therefore more susceptible to oxidation by light, especially as many of them are more deeply coloured than monoterpenes. Conversely, monoterpenes are more likely to oxidize in the presence of oxygen in air, although oxygen does play a part in producing other functional groups (see below).

Diterpenes   Diterpenes consist of two monoterpenes, i.e. four isoprene units, and are found to a much lesser extent in essential oils as they are bigger, heavier, less volatile molecules. Therapeutically, diterpenes have a weak anti-infective action, being antibacterial, antiviral and antifungal in some cases; they are also slightly expectorant and are thought to balance the endocrine system.

There are also terpenoid molecules that consist of six or even eight iso-prene units, but these are much too heavy to evaporate during the extraction process, and so they are not found in essential oils. This group includes steroids and some hormones.

Other constituents As discussed above, terpenes are all made up of a number of isoprene units, or multiples of *five* carbon atoms (with a minimum of two), in a *chain* (called aliphatic molecules). When *six* carbon atoms combine in a *ring* this is known as a benzene or aromatic ring, or, more commonly now, as a hydrocarbon phenyl ring. With either a chain or a ring formation, other functional groups of atoms may attach themselves to form molecules with a variety of shapes, and therefore with different therapeutic properties. Where molecules consist of only hydrogen and carbon they are called unsubstituted hydrocarbons (i.e. monoterpenes, sesquiterpenes and diterpenes), but when other functional groups attach themselves, some of the hydrogen atoms are replaced with oxygen and these are termed sub-stituted compounds. Terpenoid alcohols, aldehydes, ketones and acids are formed when groups of atoms attach to chain molecules. Phenolic com-pounds are formed when these same functional groups attach to a phenyl ring, with the addition of another group of molecules called phenols.

Terpenic alcohols Terpenic alcohols are formed when an aliphatic terpene chain is joined by an unstable hydroxyl group (water molecules that have lost one of the hydrogen atoms), and may be monoterpenols, sesquiter-penols or diterpenols according to the size of the aliphatic chain to which they become attached. The suffix '-ol' is helpful in identifying the alco-hols, although confusion may arise as many phenols also end in 'ol'. The change in shape that occurs as a result of the addition of the hydroxyl group will denote the characteristics, both chemical and therapeutic, of the individual compound, with some remaining in a linear chain and others becoming cyclic. The aroma of essential oils with a high proportion of alcohols in them tends to be associated with flowers and to be a pleasant gentle smell such as rose or geranium.

Monoterpenols Monoterpenols are most commonly found in essential oils and include geraniol (in palmarosa), linalol (in lavender and neroli), ter-pineol-4-ol (in large quantities in tea tree oil) and citronellol (in rose and geranium). They are strong anti-infective agents, being antibacterial and antiviral. There are many reports on the use of essential oils against infec-tions of various pathologies, but most of these have investigated the use of whole essential oils. It is difficult, therefore, to attribute their effectiveness specifically to monoterpenols, particularly as it may be the synergistic blend of a variety of constituents that affects the infective organisms. Watt (personal communication, 1996) suggests that it is not sufficient simply to quote the Latin name of an essential oil and expect to obtain a standard product: he quotes the example of *Melaleuca alternifolia* (tea tree) as an antiviral and antibacterial agent, several subvarieties of which are used as tea tree oil, and recommends that the best anti-infective properties come from *Melaleuca*, terpinen-4-ol type. Monoterpenols are also known to be stimulating and energizing, and to have low toxicity.

Sesquiterpenols   Sesquiterpenols are formed when the hydroxyl group attaches to a sesquiterpene molecule; they are decongestant and generally toning to the body. A few sesquiterpenols are thought to act as cardiac or hepatic stimulants. An example of a sesquiterpenol is farnesol, found in frankincense.

Diterpenols   Diterpenols, like diterpenes, are heavier than their mono- or sesqui- counterparts, making them less volatile, so they are less frequently found in essential oils. Chemically they are similar in structure to human steroids and consequently can potentially help in balancing the endocrine system; an example is sclareol found in clary sage.

Aldehydes   Aldehydes are formed when carbon atoms are joined by a hydrogen atom and a carboxyl group (carbon and oxygen linked by a double bond) but are not within a carbonic chain. However, the double bond means that aldehydes can break down relatively easily so will oxidize quickly, and this process is self-catalysing. As oxidation occurs, aldehydes are converted to acids which can be astringent and often act as a catalyst for other reactions.

It is important, therefore, to store and blend essential oils containing significant amounts of aldehydes with care. If an aromatherapist is considering adding essential oils to soaps, those that contain mainly alcohols rather than aldehydes should be selected as the latter will react with the alkaline nature of the soap to form salts such as sodium benzoate.

Aldehydes tend to smell quite sharp; for example, the aroma of almonds in sweet almond oil is due to the presence of benzyl aldehyde, which is also responsible for the rapid oxidation that can occur with this base oil. It is worth noting that approximately 1% of the population is allergic to benzyl aldehyde, and that there is about 1–2% benzyl aldehyde in sweet almond oil. This is a relatively small amount but it would be good practice to question clients about possible allergy to almonds if the therapist intends to use sweet almond as a carrier oil.

Some aldehydes are not terpenic, i.e. they are not made up of isoprene units, and, due to the presence of additional double bonds, are even more reactive than terpenic aldehydes, e.g. cinnamic aldehyde in cinnamon oil, which oxidizes readily to cinnamic acid.

Many of the aldehydes are skin irritants or sensitizers, so care should be taken when administering any oil with a high aldehyde content. This is especially so in the case of citral, which is found in bergamot, melissa and the citrus oils. The effects are worse, however, when the aldehyde is isolated from the whole essential oil. Aldehydes also have a sedative action and are generally calming, acting as a nerve tonic and reducing blood pressure and temperature. Certain aldehydes possess strong antiseptic properties, being antifungal, antiviral and antibacterial. In addition they can be used as anti-inflammatory agents.

Aldehydes are easily recognized as all the names end either in 'aldehyde' or in 'al', as in citronellal, geranial and neral.

Esters   When an acid and an alcohol combine, esters, together with water are formed; some are terpenoid, others non-terpenoid. They tend to have fruity pleasant aromas, and their names usually have the suffix 'ate', e.g. linalyl acetate found in clary sage oil. They have a mild action, are anti-inflammatory, calming and sedative, have a balancing action, and seem to possess antispasmodic properties.

The chemical reaction involving water is important in aromatherapy for, if water is added to an essential oil high in esters to produce a spray (for example to camomile oil which contains about 60% esters), catalysis could occur that would reduce the amount and therefore the effects of the esters, but increase the proportion of acids and/or alcohols in the blend. It is thus recommended that any product involving water and ester-rich essential oils is used immediately and then discarded.

Ketones   A carboxyl group (oxygen plus carbon with a double bond) within a carbonic chain results in a ketone being formed. Ketones normally have the letters 'one' at the end of the name (camphor is an exception) and may be terpenic or non-terpenic.

Ketones have a valuable role to play in therapy for respiratory tract infections as they are expectorant and mucolytic, and are also cytophylactic. However, oils containing ketones should be used with care for some, such as thujone, found particularly in sage, thuja and pennyroyal oils, are known to be abortifacient if used to excess. Thujone is a terpenic ketone with two isomer forms, α and β, with the α isomer being the more toxic (Tisserand & Balacs 1995, p. 200). Watt (personal communication, 1996) states that the α isomer may be as much as four times more toxic than the β, and that it is therefore not possible to make a broad claim that all thujone-containing oils are toxic, without knowing which isomer exists in the oil to be used. Others can be neurotoxic when ingested, occasionally leading to epileptic fits, as in the case of pinocamphone in essential oil of hyssop. When using essential oils that contain ketones, it is wise to blend them in very low dilutions and avoid prolonged administration; ketone-containing oils are probably best identified as being contraindicated during pregnancy until more research evidence is available to demonstrate their safety.

Phenols   Phenols are formed when an alcohol hydroxyl group attaches itself to a benzene ring. Electronically, phenols are uniformly stable and strongly positive, which makes them chemically very active. Many of the names end in 'ol', which can cause confusion with alcohols, but some end in 'ole' such as fenchole in fennel oil.

Phenols are well known as strong antiseptic and antibacterial agents, and as stimulants of the immune and nervous systems. However, they are also skin irritants so they should be blended in low dilutions. Aeschbach et al (1994) found the phenols, carvacrol, thymol and 6-gingerol to have useful antioxidant properties; this was supported by research into ageing by Deans et al (1993).

Oxides   1,8-Cineole, sometimes known as eucalyptol(e), is the most commonly occurring oxide in essential oils. Chemically oxides are formed when the oxygen in a ring structure links two carbon molecules. Oxides share similarities with phenols, and should therefore be treated with the same caution in respect of skin irritation. 1,8-Cineole is a strong expectorant, mucolytic and decongestant; it is found in eucalyptus and thyme oils in large amounts, in rosemary oil and as a trace in many other oils.

Coumarins   Coumarins, a type of lactone, are what gives newmown grass its characteristic smell. They are not volatile substances and therefore are found only in essential oils obtained by solvent extraction or expression – primarily the citrus essences – rather than those extracted by steam distillation.

Furocoumarins   Furocoumarins are photosensitizers and cause the development of irregular pigmentation and potential burning if skin is exposed to the sun directly after using oils containing them. These include bergapten found in bergamot oil.

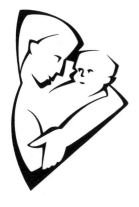

Chapter 4 # Aromatherapy-related Anatomy and Physiology

Aromatherapy is often derided by sceptics as simply the use of pleasantly smelling oils to relax people, by applying them through massage or adding them to the bath. However, it is this very attitude that potentially makes essential oils so dangerous and leaves them open to misuse or abuse through lack of knowledge. While there is much work being carried out into the effects of both the aromas on the mind and the method of administration on the body, there is also a vast exploration being made of the properties, actions and interactions of the chemical constituents of essential oils.

Research evidence is vital if aromatherapy is to be taken as a serious, credible and respectable therapy in its own right, and anecdotal accounts, although useful, are no longer sufficient to support the acquisition of sound knowledge. Practitioners must possess a thorough working knowledge and understanding of the oils, in the context in which they intend to use them, or know where to find accurate, research-based information; they should refrain from using essential oils with which they are unfamiliar until they have studied them in depth. This entails an understanding of the chemical components, the ways in which they are absorbed into the body, metabolized and excreted, as well as the possible side-effects and adverse reactions, contraindications and precautions. Comprehensive records should be maintained, both in individual case notes and centrally, to enable the identification of untoward or hitherto unrecognized reactions. At present there is no centralized system for the reporting of problems with essential oils as there is with pharmaceutical preparations.

Research into how and why essential oils work is increasing and adding to the body of professional aromatherapy knowledge. They are absorbed into the body via the skin and mucous membranes (or gastrointestinal tract if taken orally), utilized via various chemical pathways and excreted. Essential oils are fat-soluble and absorbed via cell membranes, which are rich in lipids. It is possible that they may regulate immune function by lodging in the membranes of leucocytes, or affect nerve function as do anaesthetic drugs (Balacs 1991a). The actions of essential oils may also be enhanced when administered through massage, which stimulates the circulation; damaged or diseased epidermis increases the rate of absorption into the bloodstream. Some molecules of the essential oils will also be inhaled, even when not administered directly via the respiratory tract.

As essential oils are fat-soluble they are absorbed readily into the central nervous system, for the brain is lipid-rich. They are known, from a variety of trials on both animals and humans, to affect the central nervous system, with many being sedative and others being stimulatory. α- and β-Santalol in sandalwood oil have been found to be sedative and neuroleptic but not anticonvulsant (Okugawa et al 1995), while bergamot oil appears to be both sedative and anticonvulsant (Occhiuto et al 1995). Lavender has also been shown to be anticonvulsant (Yamada et al 1994) and sedative (Karamat et al 1992). Elisabetsky et al (1995) suggest that the known hypnotic, sedative and anticonvulsant effects of linalool, found in oils such as rosewood, may act through glutamatergic transmission in the central nervous system. Conversely, sage and hyssop have a convulsant action (Millet et al 1981). Jasmine oil is known to be stimulating (Karamat et al 1992, Kikuchi et al 1989, Nakagawa et al 1992, Sugano & Sato 1991), as is rosemary (Kovar et al 1987), and sweet fennel oil may reduce mental fatigue and stress (Nagai et al 1991), as may orange (Miyazaki et al 1991, Sugano & Sato 1991).

Essential oils reach the liver via the bloodstream but pass more slowly into muscle fibres and, finally, into adipose tissue, with its slower blood flow. Here the essential oil molecules may be stored for some time, particularly terpenes which are the most fat-soluble constituents. Essential oils have been shown to have effects on the cardiovascular system, including lowering of cholesterol levels (Elson et al 1989, El Tahir et al 1993a, Gui-Yuan & Wei 1994, Hof & Ammon 1989, Kikuchi et al 1991, Nikolaevski et al 1990). Effects have also been reported on the gastrointestinal and biliary tracts (Hills & Aaronson 1991, Rees et al 1979, Trabace et al 1992). Research has also shown the actions of essential oils and/or their constituents on the respiratory tract (Aqel 1991, E1 Tahir et al 1993b, Falk-Filipsson 1993, Ferley et al 1989, Schafer & Schafer 1981, Shubina et al 1990) and the urinary tract (Eriksson & Levin 1990, Rossi et al 1988, Stanic & Samarzija 1993). Effects on other areas of the body have been demonstrated, for example on the pancreas (Al-Hader et al 1994) and the retina (Recsan et al 1997).

Essential oils, especially those containing ketones, esters and aldehydes, are thought to bind with plasma albumin. This initially reduces the overall effects of the oils on the body as the plasma albumin 'mops up' the oil molecules, but also prolongs the length of time the essential oils remain in the body. Balacs (1992c) suggests that clients with low plasma albumin levels, such as those with impaired renal or hepatic function, should be given lower doses of essential oils to avoid the risk of high circulating levels of their components.

This raises the issue of possible interactions with drugs, owing to competition for plasma albumin binding sites. Drug interactions may also occur on the surface or within cells involved in chemical metabolism, or, despite working through different mechanisms, a drug and an oil may produce similar or opposing physiological symptoms. Tisserand & Balacs (1995) consider the plasma binding mechanism to be the least likely means of drug and oil interaction as essential oil doses used in aromatherapy are insufficient to reach the circulation, but they do take into account the cellular and physiological implications. However, it is important to understand the mechanisms of metabolism of both essential oils and drugs, for if competition for plasma albumin binding sites *does* occur, the molecules of one or other substance could be left freely circulating in the blood, possibly leading to essential oils potentiating the action of the drug, or delaying or counteracting its action. One trial by Jori et al (1969) showed that certain essential oil components decreased the effects of pentobarbitol when tested in rats, which may have been due to an increase in liver enzyme activity caused by the essential oils. This would seem to indicate that the essential oils did not act directly on the same cells as the pentobarbitol, but rather exacerbated the excretion of the drug by speeding up detoxification in the liver. Transdermal penetration of drugs may be affected by essential oils and their components (Cornwell & Barry 1994, Takayama & Nagai 1994, Williams & Barry 1989), a factor to consider, for example, when treating menopausal women receiving hormone replacement therapy via skin patches.

Certain constituents of essential oils can have adverse effects if used in conjunction with specific drugs and should be avoided where a client is receiving this medication. Myristicin, a component of nutmeg oil, which may be used for women in labour (as may other oils that are contraindicated in pregnancy), is a monoamine oxidase inhibitor and should not be given orally with pethidine, although its effects when administered via other methods are not clear (Truitt et al 1963). Methyl salicylate, found in oils such as wintergreen, which should not be used in aromatherapy, but may be used in a liniment, appears to affect blood clotting times and could theoretically interact with aspirin, warfarin and heparin, although no evidence to support this is available (Le Bourhis & Soenen 1973).

Some essential oil constituents may be able to increase liver enzyme activity, as do certain drugs, implying that essential oils may exacerbate drug metabolism, although this is unlikely, given the low doses of essential oils used in aromatherapy and the consequent low levels of oils reaching the tissues. Jori et al (1969) and Kovar et al (1987) all observed increased effects with higher doses. It is therefore considered safe practice to use as low a dose as possible to achieve the desired effect; doses in pregnancy should probably not exceed 2%.

Safrole, found in cinnamon oil, in small amounts in nutmeg (up to 3%), and minutely in ylang ylang (0.03%), may cause an increase in cytochrome

P450 and other constituents may affect other enzymes (Boyland & Chasseau 1970, Parke & Rahman 1970). It enhances the effect of paracetamol, and for this reason it is probably wise to avoid using cinnamon oil in clients requiring paracetamol, as well as to advise those who have received aromatherapy treatment with cinnamon to refrain from taking the analgesic for a few hours. Oral administration of geraniol, found in geranium and rose oils, may affect liver enzymes, as do linalool, found in rosewood, and citral, a component of lemongrass and certain eucalyptus strains (Chadha & Madyastha 1984, Roffey et al 1990). 1,8-Cineole (eucalyptol), eugenol, *d*-limonene and *trans*-anethole also increase liver enzyme activity (Ariyoshi et al 1975, Jori et al 1969, Rompelberg et al 1993). Myristicin increases the activity of the detoxifying enzyme glutathione *S*-transferase and may therefore be a potential cancer chemopreventative agent (Zheng et al 1992a, 1992b). Research by Moorthy (1991) showed that pulegone, a major constituent of pennyroyal oil, which is totally contraindicated in aromatherapy, produced a 67% destruction of hepatic cytochrome P450, and a significant decrease in haem, glucose-6-phosphatase and other enzymes. Cadinene was thought to be responsible for a rise in P450 enzyme activity in Hiroi et al's work (1995). On the other hand, β-myrcene does not appear to increase drug-metabolizing enzyme activity (Madyastha & Srivatsan 1987). Other oils or their constituents reduce or inhibit liver enzyme activity, including those enzymes required for alcohol metabolism (Tisserand & Balacs 1995, p. 39)

As with drugs, the chemicals in essential oils need to be metabolized and detoxified to aid absorption and excretion. Essential oil molecules are initially altered by oxidation, reduction or hydrolysis, mainly in the liver, but also by the lungs, intestinal mucosa, skin and plasma, depending on the route of administration. Jager et al (1992) demonstrated the presence of linalool and linalyl acetates, the main components of lavender oil, in the blood 20 minutes after dermal application of the oil; most of the oil had been eliminated from the blood within 90 minutes. The method of administration should be taken into account; for example, tests by Von Grisk & Fischer (1969) implied that rectal administration of essential oils may not be a favourable means of treating respiratory disorders. Essential oils are excreted mainly by the kidneys, and urinary content of essential oil constituents has been demonstrated by Eriksson & Levin (1990) and Parke et al (1974). Some constituents are expelled by means of respiration and some, such as citral, are utilized by the cells as energy. Falk–Filipsson (1993) found a 70% uptake of *d*-limonene following respiration, with a long half-life, suggesting that it would take about 3 days for full excretion of the chemical from the adipose tissues. On the other hand, 1,8-cineole is rapidly absorbed through inhalation, reaching a peak after about 20 minutes, but seems to have a half-life of only 10 minutes (Stimpfl et al 1995). Melzig & Teuscher (1991) postulate that there may be some pharmacological effects of inhaled essential oils via the interaction between the vascular endothelium and the olfactory nerves of the nasal mucosa. Alcohols and aldehydes, which have small molecules, are excreted faster than terpenes; molecules that bind to plasma albumin will be excreted more slowly. This may have implications for the use of essential oils in pregnancy when renal filtration is altered and larger molecules are filtered through into the urine more readily. It is interesting to note that garlic ingestion in a controlled trial of women undergoing amniocentesis significantly altered the odour of the amniotic fluid, suggesting diffusion of essential oils across the placenta (Mennella et al 1995).

The physiology of olfaction

The sense of smell is extremely sensitive in human beings, although it is far from perfect. It is possible to detect over 100 000 odours, some in concentrations of up to one in 30 billion (Carola et al 1992, p. 472), although some odours such as certain noxious gases cannot be detected.

Olfaction is classified as one of the special senses, with odour perception being transmitted directly to the brain via the first cranial nerve. High in the nasal cavity is the olfactory epithelium which contains the olfactory receptors or neurons, with a life of about 30 days; the supporting or sustentacular cells; and the basal cells, which divide to replace degenerating receptor and supporting cells.

For an aroma to be detected, the molecules of the substance must be volatile; in aromatherapy, volatile essential oil molecules pervade the air and some enter the nostrils and are picked up by the cilia at the vesicular end of the olfactory receptors. The cilia are surrounded by fluid secreted from the supporting cells and the olfactory (Bowman's) glands, in which the aromatic molecules dissolve prior to stimulation of the receptor sites. The research of Kobal et al (1992) found that aromas were processed differently according to which nostril the molecules entered, a fact that may be due to pleasant and unpleasant smells being processed by different hemispheres of the brain. This would seem to be borne out by the research of Lorig et al (1993) in which olfaction 'labelling' appears to be attributed to the left frontal brain.

The 'message' of the aroma is transmitted along the axons of the receptor cells to join other axons as part of the olfactory nerve, the fibres of which pass through the cribriform plate of the ethmoid bone in the roof of the nose to reach the olfactory bulb in the cerebrum. The olfactory bulb is actually an appendage of the brain and the axons of the neurons synapse with dendrites of other cells to form the olfactory glomeruli. The olfactory impulses are sorted in the glomeruli and pass into the olfactory tract, which passes directly to the primary cortex in the cerebrum (Fig. 4.1). Research collaboration between Germany and the UK has shown a possible trigeminal nerve involvement as well as the olfactory nerve activity (Kobal et al 1992).

Much work is being done on the effects of essential oil odours on the brain, and psychoaromatherapy is a growing field. Worwood (1990, p. 82) suggests that some essential oils stimulate the logical right side of the brain, while others stimulate the left side, a theory that is gaining credibility. When one considers the effects of the chemical components in pharmaceutical

Fig. 4.1. *(a) Diagram showing the olfactory receptors and passage of odours to the olfactory bulb. (b) Relationship of olfactory bulb and nerves to the nose, palate and brain.*

(a)

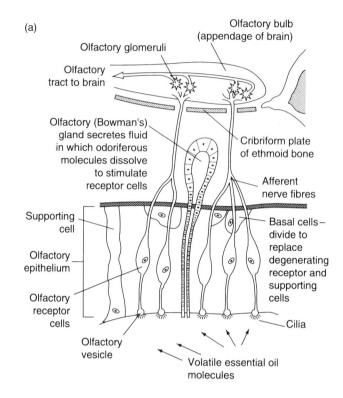

(b)

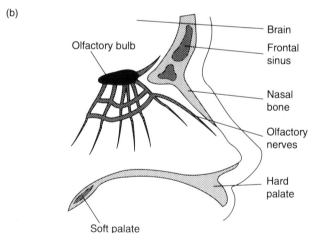

drugs, it is hardly surprising that those in essential oils should have physiologically induced effects on the psyche.

Japanese research found that machine operators' efficiency improved by 21% when the atmosphere was scented with lavender, by 33% when jasmine was used and by 54% with lemon; subsequently an environmental fragrancing system has been developed to help increase productivity (Kallan 1991).

The effects of odours on mood, creativity and perceived health have also been investigated (Knasko 1992). This work showed that mood can be adversely affected by unpleasant odours with a corresponding effect on performance, and that fresh clean smells such as lemon result in perceptions of better health, while Smith et al (1992) found that aroma could act as a contextual cue for the retrieval of verbal stimuli.

Gender differences were found in relation to the psychological impact of aromas by Takeuchi et al (1991), and Nagai et al (1991) demonstrated the value of odours in reducing fatigue and mental stress. Concentration and attention span may also be affected by aromas (Miyaki et al 1991b, Warm & Dember 1990, Warm et al 1991).

Slow brain waves, known as contingent negative variation, measured by electroencephalography, have been assessed to identify whether a selection of essential oils have the sedative or stimulant properties presumed by aromatherapists (Manley 1993). The oils achieved the expected responses and included basil, bergamot, camomile, geranium, lemon, marjoram, neroli, patchouli, peppermint, rose, rosewood and sandalwood.

Similarly, locomotor activity of the brains of mice was shown to increase after administration of rosemary oil (Kovar et al 1987), and physiological responses to peppermint oil during sleep demonstrated significant differences between odour and non-odour periods, leading the researchers to postulate that 'relaxing' aromas may enhance sleep (Badia et al 1990). Neurodepressive effects were observed in mice and rats given two varieties of Spanish mint (Perez Raya et al 1990) and in mice who received oral *Lavandula augustifolia* oil (Guillemain et al 1989). The sedative effects of lavender oil have also been demonstrated by Buchbauer et al (1991) and by Imberger and co-workers (1993), together with the excitory action of jasmine (Karamat et al 1992), although large doses of jasmine in mice have shown it to be a central nervous system depressant (Elisha et al 1988). Camomile, which is known to be sedative, has been shown to alter negative mood ratings to more positive ratings, inducing a degree of euphoria (Roberts & Williams 1992). Other oils were investigated by Santos et al (1996) and the central nervous system depression was attributed to terpenes.

In a holistic therapy such as aromatherapy it is impossible to separate the entities of body, mind and spirit, a concept that is only slowly being accepted by practitioners of conventional medicine. Psychoaromatherapy appears, however, to conform to biochemical principles and deserves much more investigation. What is, for some, even more difficult to understand is the notion that both the human body and essential oils, together with other organic substances, possess subtle energies that are capable of interacting. In a textbook aimed at exploring contemporary knowledge in relation to the use of essential oils for childbearing women, it is not feasible to discuss in depth the concept of potential subtle energies that may exist, for this is a relatively newly recognized area in Western clinical aromatherapy (although its origins are ancient), and readers are referred to the bibliography for further information.

Anatomy of the skin and the physiology of touch

The skin is the largest organ in the body, occupying over 2 m², and is part of the integumentary system. Some areas of the body are covered with very thick skin, such as the middle of the back, while other parts, for example the eyelids, have a very thin covering. Skin acts as a protective cover for the internal organs, and prevents body fluids from being lost and harmful substances such as microorganisms from gaining entry. It is virtually waterproof, but allows the passage of certain molecules, including therapeutic essential oils as well as harmful chemicals. When the body is warm, temperature control is achieved by means of the excretion of sweat, which cools on exposure to air, as well as by vasodilation and heat radiation; on cold days vasoconstriction in the skin acts as an insulating mechanism to retain body heat. Excretion of some waste materials such as urea and nitrogen occurs via the skin; and useful ultraviolet rays convert 7-dehydrocholesterol into vitamin D, while harmful ultraviolet light is screened out by the skin. Finally, the skin is an important sensory organ (see below).

The outer layer of skin, the epidermis, has no blood vessels but, as it is very thin, most cuts and abrasions penetrate the dermal layer beneath and so draw blood. Within the epidermis there are between three and five layers, depending on the thickness of the skin, starting with the stratum corneum and ending with the stratum spinosum and stratum basale, these latter two being cumulatively known as the stratum germinativum as they generate new cells. In addition, the palms of the hands and the soles of the feet contain the stratum lucidum and the stratum granulosum.

The stratum corneum consists of parallel rows of dead cells of soft keratin to maintain the skin's elasticity and to protect the living cells beneath from drying out due to exposure to the air. The dead cells are constantly being shed and replaced by cells pushed up from the germinative layer below. The palms and soles have the stratum lucidum next, which is also made up of dead cells and acts as an ultraviolet light filter to prevent sunburning of the areas. The stratum granulosum beneath the stratum lucidum contains granules of keratohyaline, which is needed for the process of keratinization or cell death. The stratum spinosum serves as a support and binding, and facilitates the process of protein synthesis leading to cell division and growth. The stratum basale divides the epidermis from the dermis and also helps to produce new cells to replace those lost at the surface.

The dermis or 'true' skin is a strong connective mesh of thick protein collagen fibres to make the skin tough, thinner but strong supporting reticular fibres, and elastic fibres to provide flexibility. The dermis also contains blood vessels, which carry the fat-soluble essential oil molecules around the body, lymphatic vessels, nerve fibres, glands and hair follicles, and is indefinably divided into a papillary and a reticular layer.

The papillary layer of loose connective tissue with bundles of collagenous fibres has tiny finger-like papillae that join it to the epidermal ridges.

The papillae contain capillaries to nourish the epidermis as well as the special touch receptors called Meissner's corpuscles. The reticular layer of dense connective tissue has a mesh of collagenous fibre bundles forming a strong elastic network with a dominant directional pattern in different areas of the body. Tension lines in the skin resulting from the directional pattern of the fibres are called Langer's or cleavage lines; surgical incisions made parallel to the cleavage lines lead to more rapid healing and less scarring. Overstretching of the dermis during pregnancy can lead to tearing of the collagen and elastic fibres, with the repairing scar tissue resulting in striae gravidarum. Also within the reticular layer are blood and lymphatic vessels, nerves and free nerve endings, fat cells, sebaceous glands and hair roots. Pacinian corpuscles, or deep pressure receptors, are also found within this layer and in the subcuticular hypodermal layer. Muscle fibres are present as well in the reticular layer of the genital area and nipples.

The subcutaneous hypodermis of loose fibrous connective tissue is thick and has a rich supply of blood vessels, lymphatics and nerves as well as the bases of the hair follicles and sweat glands. In some parts of the body such as the breasts there are also thick layers of adipose cells (Fig. 4.2).

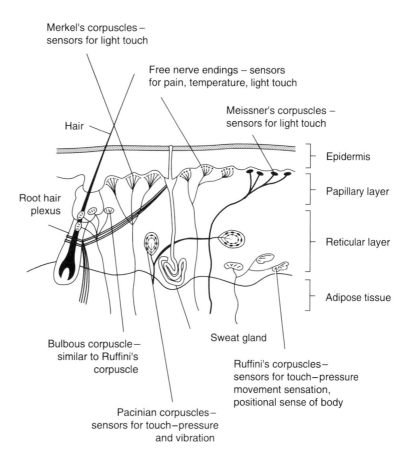

Fig. 4.2. *Diagram showing sensory receptors in the skin.*

Merkel's corpuscles – sensors for light touch

Free nerve endings – sensors for pain, temperature, light touch

Meissner's corpuscles – sensors for light touch

Hair

Epidermis

Papillary layer

Root hair plexus

Reticular layer

Adipose tissue

Bulbous corpuscle – similar to Ruffini's corpuscle

Sweat gland

Ruffini's corpuscles – sensors for touch–pressure movement sensation, positional sense of body

Pacinian corpuscles – sensors for touch–pressure and vibration

Sensory reception of the skin   A variety of sensations are perceived by the skin owing to the presence of sensory receptors, and in fact the sense of touch, once thought to be one sense, is actually a response to three stimuli: pressure, temperature and pain. Light touch without deformity of the skin surface is detected in the dermis by the free nerve endings and Meissner's corpuscles and in the epidermis of the palms and soles by free nerve endings and Merkel's corpuscles. Deep pressure results in the skin surface being temporarily deformed and is detected by Pacinian corpuscles or mechanoreceptors which measure pressure changes, situated in the dermis and subcutaneous layer of the skin. Variable vibrations of the skin are detected by Pacinian corpuscles, Meissner's corpuscles and corpuscles of Ruffini, depending on the frequency of vibration. Naked nerve endings can measure heat and cold, while specialized free nerve endings throughout the body are receptive to different types of pain. Continuous low-key stimulation of slow-conducting nerve fibres, mainly in the superficial layers of the skin, is thought to be the mechanism by which itches and ticklish sensations are perceived. The sensory neural pathways to the brain for both light touch and pain are situated in the spinothalamic tract ending in the cerebral cortex, and it is for this reason that effleurage (light massage) can act as a means of easing pain.

Aromatherapists constantly debate the issue of whether essential oils work because of their chemical constituents or because of the method of administration, especially massage. There is an increasing amount of research into this area and into the ability of essential oil molecules to be absorbed by the skin. Jager and co-workers' (1992) trial using lavender oil in a massage showed constituents of the oil in the blood only 5 minutes after administration; they reached a peak at 20 minutes and were removed from the blood by 90 minutes. Weyers & Brodbeck (1989) tested the amounts of 1,8-cineole in skeletal muscle following dermal application of eucalyptus and found significant differences according to the method of application. There was a 320% greater bioavailability of 1,8-cineole when an applicator was used compared with an occlusive dressing.

Massage is thought to increase the rate of systemic absorption of essential oils due to the increased blood flow. However, while it might be expected that a warm room, warm client and warm hands of the aromatherapist could increase absorption of the oils, it is probable that the molecules are more readily vaporized and are thus inhaled to take effect in the body. The most permeable areas of the skin for the passage of essential oil molecules are the palms of the hands and the soles of the feet, the forehead, scalp, axillae and, probably impractically, the scrotum. The legs, abdomen and trunk are less permeable but hirsute areas of the body facilitate the passage of molecules as they travel along the hair shaft to the dermal layer. Mucous membranes are highly permeable and essential oils should not be applied to these areas except in extremely low dilutions, as the area may become severely irritated.

The carrier oil used will also affect the rate of absorption, with many of the thicker more viscous carriers impairing the rate, although those rich in polyunsaturates will be absorbed fairly quickly. However, volatility of the essential oil molecules may be decreased by a particular carrier, thereby affecting the absorption rate, or skin enzymes may begin the process of metabolism of the molecules as happens with certain esters, notably benzyl acetate (Balacs 1992b). Nevertheless, a group of skin enzymes called P450s which help to detoxify poisons, making them more water soluble prior to urinary excretion, may chemically alter some essential oils, in some cases producing toxins. This is known to be the case with pennyroyal, an essential oil completely contraindicated in aromatherapy, and may be responsible for the toxicity of other essential oils. This effect is significant for clients taking certain medications, for example lipid-lowering agents, steroids and anti-epileptic drugs such as phenobarbitone, in whom the drug's increased P450 activity could increase essential oil metabolism (Balacs 1992b).

Physiology of respiration

Inhalation of essential oil molecules plays a part in every aromatherapy treatment. Even when the method of administration is via the skin, some of the molecules will pervade the air and a few will enter the nostrils, passing directly to the brain to be perceived as an aroma, and affecting cerebral processes such as mood. Molecules also travel into the nasopharynx, the trachea and thence to the lungs, via the bronchi.

Within the lungs the bronchi divide further and further into a 'respiratory tree' and finally into respiratory bronchioles ending in the microscopic air sacs, or alveoli, in which gaseous exchange occurs. Each lung contains over 350 million alveoli bunched in grape-like clusters, surrounded by capillaries. The alveolar and capillary walls are extremely thin to allow for the diffusion of oxygen and carbon dioxide between them. Once in the blood vessels oxygen and any other molecules carried with it are transported partially in solution and partially with haemoglobin around the body to be used as required.

It is obvious that, for some conditions involving the cardiorespiratory system, administration of essential oils by inhalation will be the treatment of choice, although Ryman (1991, p. viii) states this as her preferred route for almost all clients. It is also possible that certain components of the oils possess a particular affinity for specific organs in the body. Falk–Filipsson (1993), for example, suggests that monoterpenes are very soluble in blood, have a high respiratory uptake and are easily stored in adipose tissues, and showed an approximately 70% pulmonary uptake of *d*-limonene after inhalation.

The absorption of essential oil molecules through inhalation and the effect of the fragrances on cerebral activity is not dependent on aroma perception. This has been shown by the work of Nasel et al (1994) in which inhalation of 1,8-cineole by nine subjects (including one anosmic person) demonstrated similar effects on the general cerebral blood flow of all nine subjects. The authors postulated that inhalation of essential oils may have a direct pharmacological action on the brain, a fact that is increasingly being used to improve work efficiency and productivity (Sugano & Sato 1991). This is further borne out by the increased attention span, concentration and efficiency that occurred, irrespective of personal like or dislike of aromas, in the early work of Tasev et al (1969), although Kikuchi and colleagues (1989) found that aroma preference did improve performance. Other work on human reaction times after inhalation of various essential oils has also been carried out (Karamat et al 1992, Miyake et al 1991, Miyaki et al 1991b, Sugano 1989).

In practice it is generally felt that many effects, and specifically relaxation, are the result of a combination of inhalation and dermal absorption of essential oil molecules, massage and the accompanying rest and nurturing by the therapist. Wilkinson's (1995) trial using massage alone or massage with essential oils on patients with terminal cancer did show a statistically significant difference in the aromatherapy group, in terms of relaxation and reduction of stress.

Summary

This chapter has specifically covered aspects of aromatherapy-related anatomy and physiology. Readers who do not possess a comprehensive knowledge and understanding of the anatomy and physiology related to pregnancy and childbirth should refer to *Mayes' Midwifery* (1997), edited by Sweet with Tiran. Where appropriate, a brief explanation of physiological changes is included in this book in Chapter 7, 'Using Essential Oils in Maternity Care'.

Chapter 5 # Safety of Essential Oils in Pregnancy and Childbirth

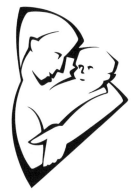

The issue of safety of essential oils concerns all aromatherapists, but the specific problem of identifying which oils are safe to use in childbearing women is one that is still very much open to question. It is necessary first to consider general safety data available on essential oils and then to apply the principles to pregnancy, childbirth, lactation and the neonate.

Certain essential oils are completely contraindicated in aromatherapy because of their toxicity (Box 5.1). Others have uses only in perfumery rather than therapeutic aromatherapy. The main factors that govern the use of an essential oil for therapeutic use are photoxicity, dermal and oral toxicity, carcinogenicity and general pharmacological effects. In maternity care the issues centre around teratogenicity, mutagenicity, oils that are

Box 5.1	Hazardous essential oils contraindicated in aromatherapy
Armoise (mugwort)	Horseradish
Arnica	Jaborandi leaf
Basil (exotic)	Melilotus
Birch (sweet)	Mustard
Bitter almond	Origanum
Boldo leaf	Pennyroyal
Broom	Pine (dwarf)
Buchu	Rue
Calamus	Sassafras
Camphor (brown or yellow)	Savin
Cassia	Savory (summer)
Chervil	Tansy
Cinnamon bark	Thuja
Clove (bud, leaf or stem)	Tonka
Costus	Vanilla
Deertongue	Wintergreen
Elecampane	Wormwood
Fennel (bitter)	

emmenagoguic or abortifacient, and an understanding of how the physiology of pregnancy and the pharmacology of essential oils interact.

Practitioners attempting to elicit information about safety of essential oils in pregnancy will find a plethora of conflicting and confusing advice, especially in books aimed at the consumer. Indeed, some readily available books for pregnant women contain misleading and occasionally potentially dangerous information. One of the main aromatherapy texts on safety (International School of Aromatherapy 1993) suggests, correctly, that many other substances may adversely affect the fetus, for example alcohol, but fails to take into account the amount of research supporting this fact. In aromatherapy there is virtually no research into the effects on the fetus of essential oils administered to the mother during pregnancy. What little work has been carried out on expectant women *assumes* a degree of safety of the oils being used, merely through lack of evidence to the contrary. It is therefore vital that professionals using essential oils for expectant, labouring and newly delivered mothers and their infants err on the side of caution until more data are available.

Phototoxicity

Certain essential oils are known to possess some phototoxic effects but the degree of the reaction is unknown in many oils. The information that is available has resulted from extensive testing of animals, but it is recognized that there are differences between the physiologies of the various animals tested and human physiology. Consequently the information can only be considered a guide until further research has been carried out. Of significance to those caring for pregnant women are the potential effects on the skin of essential oils known to cause photosensitivity at a time when there are raised melanocytic hormone levels circulating in the body. The citrus oils are generally quoted as having some degree of phototoxicity, which is of relevance in maternity care, for these are otherwise considered to be among the safest oils to use during pregnancy. Research in 1985 by Naganuma et al demonstrated the active phototoxic ingredients of lemon oil samples from around the world to be mainly the furanocoumarins bergapten and to some extent oxypeucedanin, with the latter component also being found in samples of lime and bitter orange essence. However Tisserand & Balacs (1995, p. 86) suggest that distilled lemon and lime oils, and expressed mandarin, tangerine and sweet orange oils, are not phototoxic.

Cases of skin reactions, including one requiring admission to a burns unit, have been reported following the use of bergamot-containing suntan lotion (Meyer 1970). This author has had experience of adverse reaction with lime juice. The son of a friend living in Australia was playing under lime trees and became covered in juice from the fruit. A combination of the hot sun and the lime juice caused severe burns to his body that necessitated hospital admission; treatment was delayed because the staff did not recognize the skin lesions as burns as they were unaware of the potential harm of lime juice in the sun. The boy now has several scars on his body.

Phototoxicity should not be a problem if doses are kept below 2%, but in high summer it may be wise to advise women who have received massage with bergamot and lemon oils to avoid direct exposure of the skin to sunlight for about 2 hours, particularly those women for whom facial chloasma is already a problem, as it indicates higher than normal circulating levels of melanocytic hormone.

Dermal toxicity

Irritation of the skin has been reported on many occasions in relation to several different essential oils (Box 5.2), although this does seem to be dose related. Allergy to camomile oil has been recorded (McGeorge & Steele 1991, Van Ketel 1987), and a case of chemical burns resulting from contact with neat peppermint oil was reported by Parys (1983). Allergy to both dermal and oral application of tea tree oil was found to be due to the presence of 1,8-cineole (De Groot & Weyland 1993) although Southwell et al (1997) found skin irritancy to be no worse in tea tree oils with high levels of 1,8-cineole than in those with lower levels. They attributed dermal irritancy of tea tree oil to aromadendrene, a sesquiterpene. However, 1,8-cineole may be the cause of similar irritation to eucalyptus oil (Spoerke et al 1989), while benzoin has long been known to cause allergic reactions in sensitive individuals (Cullen et al 1974, James et al 1984, Mann 1982, Rademaker & Kirby 1987, Tripathi et al 1990).

The issue of whether the aromatherapist could develop dermatitis from frequent use of different oils is important. Certainly there are anecdotal reports from therapists about the effects on their hands; this author experiences itching after using camomile and a colleague is unable to use lavender oil for the same reason. Occupational allergy to lavender oil has also been reported in a hairdresser (Brandao 1986); French marigold (tagetes) has resulted in eczematous rashes in one practitioner (Bilsland & Strong 1990); and prolonged exposure to peppermint oil, an ingredient in several dental preparations, caused hypersensitivity in a dental technician (Dooms-Goossens et al 1977). Selvaag et al (1995) reported the case of an aromatherapist who developed eczema on her arms, trunk, legs, hands and face and who was found, following patch-testing, to be sensitive to 17 out of

---

Box 5.2 Essential oils that may cause adverse skin reactions

Basil (French)	Jasmine?
Benzoin	Lavender
Bergamot	Lemon
Cedarwood (Virginian)	Lemongrass
Camomile (German, Roman)	Melissa
Cinnamon (leaf)	Orange (sweet?)
Citronella	Peppermint
Geranium (especially Bourbon)	Tea tree
Ginger (in high concentrations)	Thyme

the 20 essential oils that she used in her practice, with lemongrass oil being the primary sensitizing agent.

On some occasions the allergy may be due to a single chemical component of an oil, but as that component may be present in many different oils in varying proportions it is necessary to elicit the precise chemical cause. Hyperplasia of sebaceous glands following topical application of citral (in rats) has been recorded (Sandbank et al 1988). Geraniol, a common constituent of several oils, has been shown to lead to dermatitis (Cardullo et al 1989, Guerra et al 1987), and sensitivity to *d*-limonene (in lemon and lemongrass oils) was reported in a barman who frequently handled lemon slices to add to drinks (Audicana & Bernaola 1994). It was suggested that people who frequently came into contact with citrus fruit (and, by implication, citrus oils?) should be regularly patch-tested for sensitivity. Cinnamon leaf may also cause irritation (Calnan 1976).

There are accounts of skin complaints arising from the extended use of an essential oil or a substance containing an essential oil (Sharma et al 1987), but this should not be a problem for clients receiving professional aromatherapy as it is generally believed that no single oil should be used continuously for more than 3 weeks. Contact dermatitis has also been reported following inhalation of vapours of a tea tree oil infusion (De Groot 1996). In another case, prolonged use of aroma lamps for diffusion of essential oils to allow inhalation of the vapours caused such severe resistant and relapsing eczema that complete interior decoration of the patient's home became necessary (Schaller & Korting 1995). Self-medication with commercially available tea tree preparation applied neat has also resulted in several cases of skin irritation (Knight & Haussen 1994).

The quality of an essential oil should be taken into account when considering the possibility of dermal toxicity, for the pure organic oils should not be contaminated. Oxidation and ageing may also trigger skin reactions, so it is wise to discard oils that are past their recommended shelf-life. Research in 1969 by Woeber & Krombach supported the use of pure, good quality, non-oxidized oils and suggested that the substances produced in the extraction process of some low-grade essential oils could act as skin sensitizers. Rudski and colleagues (1976) investigated sensitivity to 35 essential oils and found that, as well as those expected to cause reactions such as bitter orange, bergamot, geranium and eucalyptus, others including ylang ylang, cedarwood and citronella gave positive results.

Experiments on rabbits have led to the production of monographs by the Research Institute of Fragrance Materials (RIFM) as a guide to dermal sensitivity; these are used by the perfumery and food industries and by aromatherapists. Nevertheless the RIFM recognizes the need for additional research as there are differences in the rates of skin absorption between rabbits and humans, and the monographs can only be used as a guide.

Japanese research is cited in one of the safety guides available (International School of Aromatherapy 1993, p. 12) in which a large-scale study of 200 volunteers over 8 years using well over a quarter of a million patch tests identified certain factors regarding skin sensitivity to essential oils. These included the facts that men were more sensitive than women and that sensitivity in many subjects was increased around the time of change of season. Of significance to pregnant and childbearing women is the observation that illness and stressful situations – including pregnancy – resulted in a greater degree of skin sensitivity than normal.

Oral toxicity

Essential oils are administered orally by medically qualified aromatherapists in Europe, notably France, as an alternative or complement to conventional pharmaceutical preparations. Jean Valnet is the contemporary leading authority on the gastrointestinal administration of essential oils. Some aromatherapy books, including those for the consumer, advocate the use of small amounts of essential oils in cookery. While it is perfectly probable that essential oils may be both pleasant and safe to use in this way, clinical aromatherapists in the UK do not prescribe essential oils orally unless the practitioner is very experienced. It is not possible to monitor the rate of absorption via the intestinal mucosa, and insufficient is known about the changes that may occur to essential oils in the gut although effects of essential oils on gastrointestinal muscle, e.g. peppermint, are well known (Dew et al 1984, Hills & Aaronson 1991, Leicester & Hunt 1982, Taddei et al 1988).

Tisserand & Balacs (1995, p. 235) advocate extreme caution if essential oils are administered orally to pregnant women; it is the recommendation of this author that, until more evidence is available to demonstrate safety, oral use of concentrated essential oils is totally avoided during pregnancy.

There are some reports of poisoning from the ingestion of large amounts of essential oils such as citronella (Temple et al 1991) and eucalyptus (Gurr & Scroggie 1965, Spoerke et al 1989). A 2-year-old who ingested up to 10 ml of oil of cloves became comatose, acidotic and severely hypoglycaemic, and acute liver damage and disseminated intravascular coagulation followed. As the symptoms were similar to those in cases of paracetamol overdoses, similar treatment was given and eventually the boy made a full recovery. It was noted that the chemical metabolic pathways normally utilized by the components of oils of cloves became oversaturated, necessitating the utilization of alternative pathways in the body (Hartnoll et al 1993). However, in a review of 41 cases of eucalyptus oil poisoning in Queensland, Australia, there were no fatalities, even in children who had drunk up to 45 ml of the oil (Webb & Pitt 1993). Some therapeutic work has, however, been done with essential oils in capsule form, for example peppermint (Somerville et al 1984) and garlic (Joshi et al 1987).

For pregnant women the culinary use of herbs enables them to receive the therapeutic effects of the plant without the concentration of essential oils administered in other ways; neither will it lead to potential gastric irritation or uncertain absorption rate of ingesting essential oils. However,

Bakerink et al (1996) recorded two separate cases in which Hispanic children were given a traditional mint tea to treat minor ailments, which was subsequently found to contain pennyroyal. One child developed liver dysfunction and epileptic encephalopathy, while the other child died as a result of hepatic failure and cerebral necrosis.

From a safety viewpoint it is vital that essential oils are stored out of reach of children and that any blends given to women for home use are labelled 'not for internal use'. If accidental ingestion does occur, the general practitioner should be called or the person taken to hospital, especially if he or she becomes symptomatic; an emergency ambulance should be called if there is loss of consciousness. It is vital to inform the medical team of the precise oil taken and the amount, where this is known; the Poisons Unit at Guy's Hospital in London may be able to advise doctors as to the most appropriate treatment. Traditionally gastric lavage is used to empty the stomach, but practitioners should not attempt to induce vomiting or use emetic agents without expert advice. Pilapil (1989) reports the case of a child who ingested cinnamon oil who suffered a range of symptoms, including virtual coma. Milk was given orally to neutralize stomach acidity and then ipecacuanha to induce vomiting, followed by activated charcoal; complete recovery was made within 5 hours. Activated charcoal was also used effectively to treat a small boy who had drunk 10 ml of tea tree oil (Jacobs & Hornfeldt 1994); Beccara (1995) details a similar case. There is one recorded case of accidental ingestion of camphorated oil in a pregnant woman at term (Weiss & Catalano 1973) who developed grand mal seizures and required gastric lavage. The baby was born the following day, and although he did smell of camphor (as did the amniotic fluid), no signs of physical abnormality were noticed. However, as maternal detoxification is more effective than that of neonates it was suggested that similar cases may benefit from delaying delivery of the baby. The author cited a previous case of camphor ingestion which caused pregnancy complications and neonatal death.

Carcinogenicity

Little information is available regarding the potential carcinogenic and cytotoxic effects of essential oils. Those oils recognized to have a strong possibility of being carcinogenic, including camphor, sassafras and calamus, are already contraindicated in aromatherapy (International School of Aromatherapy 1993, pp. 93–95). The dangers of these essential oils are due to the high levels of safrole, but it would perhaps be wise to refrain from using any oil containing safrole in pregnancy; this includes cinnamon and nutmeg. Basil is also thought to have a potential carcinogenic effect if used in large doses (Anthony 1987, Zangouras et al 1981).

It would appear that more work is being carried out on the anticancer effects of essential oils than on the tumour-inducing effects (de la Puerta et al 1993, Fang et al 1989, Zheng et al 1993). Interestingly, Aruna & Sivaramakrishnan (1996) investigated cumin, poppy and basil oils and found each to have some effectiveness in increasing the activity and concentration of the carcinogen detoxifying enzyme, glutathione *S*-transferase, indicating a possible use as protective agents against carcinogens. Bannerjee et al (1994) also demonstrated that a range of essential oils, including coriander, ginger, nutmeg and cumin, may affect mutagenic and carcinogenic agents, while Lam & Zheng (1991) carried out similar trials on oils such as caraway, lemongrass, clove, eucalyptus, fennel, spearmint and others. Essential oils from the Umbelliferae family, which contain myristicin, may also be protective against cancer (Zheng et al 1992a, 1992b). Onion and garlic essential oils have also been shown to inhibit tumour development (Belman 1983) and citrus oils with a substantially high level of *d*-limonene could have a part to play (Elson et al 1988, Wattenberg & Coccia 1991).

Teratogenicity and mutagenicity

The issue of possible effects of chemical substances on the embryo and fetus has become an ethicolegal minefield and a highly emotive subject. Since the disasters of thalidomide and stilboestrol the pharmaceutical industry and the general public have become increasingly aware of the potential dangers of substances entering the mother's body, particularly during the early part of pregnancy, and the litigious, blame-laying culture of the late twentieth century has fuelled these concerns, although perhaps not without some justification.

The pharmaceutical industry is required to undertake a strict programme of testing the efficacy and safety of new drugs, which commences with the need to pay several thousand pounds to the government in order to obtain the licence to begin development. Early research is conducted in vitro, then formative tests are carried out on animals. If these prove safe, healthy volunteer humans are exposed to the drugs under development before finally, in controlled experiments, the new drug is tested on a sample of the particular client group for which it is eventually intended. If, at any time, side-effects and complications prove potentially too harmful to humans, the research process is abandoned and development discontinued. This process, of course, is designed to elicit, at as early a stage as possible, any dangers or contraindications; abandonment of the programme will cost the relevant company millions of pounds. When development of a new drug is complete, a licence to sell it is granted by the government but vigilant observations for undesirable side-effects continue. Most pharmaceutical companies take a cautious stance in respect of pregnancy as there will normally be insufficient data on teratogenic and mutagenic effect apart from tests conducted on animals, or in rare reported cases in humans, usually where accidental overdoses have been taken.

With essential oils there is no legal requirement to pre-test them in the same way as drugs, although this subject has been hotly debated in the European Community, and there is no scientific evidence to support or dispute their safety during pregnancy, labour, the early puerperium or in the neonate adapting to extrauterine life. There is a wealth of anecdotal evidence in the form of women who have used various essential oils at this time, including prior to having conception confirmed. Many women become concerned that they have used essential oils during the preconception phase or the first trimester, in the same way that they worry about their consumption of alcohol, and it would indeed be inappropriate and alarmist to intimate that they have done something dangerous. However, where possible, caution in the use of essential oils at this time should be encouraged, for we do not know what effects, positive or negative, essential oils can have on the embryo and fetus.

Essential oils that appear to have caused teratogenic effect in animals have usually been administered in such high doses that comparable doses in humans would never be used, and may in fact be systemically toxic. Added to this is the difference in physiology between animals and humans, although at present the safest policy would seem to be that, where essential oils have been found to be detrimental to animal pregnancy, they should be avoided during human pregnancy.

Another factor that must be taken into account is that individual constituents of essential oils, to which various adverse effects are attributed, are not used in isolation in clinical aromatherapy; they will work synergistically with all the other components of the oil to which they belong, and any negative properties may be neutralized within the whole oil. This point can be illustrated by testing the theory that it is the high levels of sabinyl acetate in *Juniperus sabinus* and *Plecanthrus fruticosus* that are the cause of observed abortion and fetal malformation in mice. Yet in earlier work (Pages et al 1990) on *Eucalyptus globulus*, which also contains sabinyl acetate, on mice, no toxic effects on the developing embryos were found. This suggests that toxicity is related to the proportion of the relevant constituent within the individual oil.

Delgado et al (1993a, 1993b) investigated the peri-and postnatal developmental toxicity of β-myrcene, a component of juniper oil, and found that it was only with higher doses that there was significantly increased perinatal mortality, retarded postnatal development and impaired fertility in females. It was stated by the authors that comparable doses were unlikely to be attained by humans exposed to essential oils containing myrcene. Similarly, only the higher doses of citral administered orally to rats resulted in intrauterine growth retardation and some skeletal abnormalities (Nogueira et al 1995).

However, by their very nature, essential oils will cross the placental barrier, as they all have a low relative molecular mass and therefore the potential to reach the fetus. The blood–brain barrier is not well developed in the fetus, allowing substances such as essential oils to reach the fetal central nervous system where their effects are likely to be more pronounced than they would be on the maternal central nervous system. The relative immaturity of the fetal liver means that it is incapable of metabolizing a compound into a more toxic one, unlike in an adult, thus giving the fetus a degree of protection from harmful or potentially harmful constituents in essential oils. Tisserand & Balacs (1995, pp. 106–107) cite accounts of known incidents in which 1,8-cineole, safrole, myristicin, methyl salicylate and camphor have crossed the placenta to the fetus, with potential teratogenicity. They suggest that thujone-containing essential oils should be avoided during pregnancy, as thujone is convulsive and toxic to the central nervous system and nervous tissue, but dispute the necessity to withhold nutmeg oil before labour (although extreme care should be taken with its use, see individual profile in chapter 8). They also recommend that hyssop oil is contraindicated in pregnancy as it has high levels of pinocamphone and is severely neurotoxic, but is not recorded specifically as being teratogenic.

Abortifacient and emmenagogic essential oils

There is no evidence to suggest that essential oils classed as emmenagogic will also be abortifacient. However, it is probably wise, until more research has been carried out, to avoid emmenagogic oils (Box 5.3) in the first trimester of pregnancy, although a few of these may be used with caution in low dilution towards term for specific purposes, for example on the legs for oedema or via inhalation for sinus congestion. Tisserand & Balacs (1995, p. 110) argue that there is no justification for restricting essential oil use to certain specified periods during pregnancy, and that caution should be exercised throughout the antenatal phase with any oils that are potentially hazardous. It is also probably wise to limit the use of emmenagogic essential oils during the early puerperium when lochia is being discharged.

Box 5.3 Essential oils thought to be emmenagogic

Angelica	Galbanum
Aniseed (narcotic, oestrogenic)	Hyssop (moderately toxic,
Basil (?carcinogenic)	hypertensive)
Bay (narcotic)	Jasmine
Calamintha (hallucinogenic)	Juniper (abortifacient)
Caraway	Labdanum
Carrot seed	Lavender
Calendula	Marjoram
Camomile	Melissa
Cedarwood (abortifacient)	Myrrh (?toxic in large doses)
Celery seed	Nutmeg
Cinnamon leaf (hepatotoxic)	Parsley (toxic in large doses)
Citronella	Peppermint
Clary sage	Rose
Cumin	Rosemary (hypertensive)
Cypress	Sage
Fennel (narcotic, oestrogenic)	Tarragon (?carcinogenic)
Frankincense	Thyme (?toxic in large doses)

Most of the reports of fatal or near-fatal reactions to essential oils in pregnancy are related to those oils already contraindicated for therapeutic aromatherapy use. Pennyroyal, for example, is not used because of its pulegone content. Pulegone is a monoterpenic ketone that may cause serious hepatic disease or failure, so is not used for *any* client, let alone those compromised by the physiological upheaval of pregnancy. Balacs (1992a) recounts several obstetric incidents involving pennyroyal that have been reported in medical journals since the end of the nineteenth century. In some cases the women were unsuccessful in their attempts to induce abortion but suffered a variety of severe toxic effects, occasionally resulting in death.

The hepatic effects of pennyroyal have been found to be due to pulegone, isopulegone and menthofuran, although certain liver enzymes may help to metabolize pulegone to a less toxic level. When spontaneous abortion occurs with pennyroyal, or other toxic oils such as tansy or rue, it is probably as a result of maternal (rather than fetal) *poisoning*, and no proven abortifacient action can be attributed to these oils.

Research by Toaff et al in 1979, in which mice were given regular doses of citral, did not elicit toxic effects but did demonstrate a reduction in the number of ovarian follicles, ovum implantations, litter size and, consequently, successful pregnancy outcome. The adverse effects were attributed to the high doses of citral but the authors also raised questions regarding prolonged administration of lower doses of citral-containing essential oils during human pregnancy.

Essential oils with systemic effects undesirable in pregnancy

Practitioners caring for pregnant women need to be aware of the effects of any essential oil that they use in their practice, for although some may be considered acceptable in pregnancy, in that they are not abortifacient or emmenagoguic, they may cause other unwanted responses that can adversely affect either the mother or the fetus.

For example, some essential oils may cause hypertension or hypotension. Using a hypotensive oil for a women with pregnancy-induced hypertension could have the desired therapeutic effect, but this same oil would not be selected for a labouring woman in whom epidural analgesia was causing a fall in blood pressure. Essential oils considered to be hypertensives are rosemary, sage, thyme, hyssop and camphor. Sage, hyssop and camphor should, in any case, be avoided in pregnancy (see previous discussion), but thyme and especially rosemary may be used towards term, where appropriate. Oils that reduce blood pressure include clary sage, garlic, lavender, lemon, marjoram, melissa and ylang ylang. It is interesting to read that Tisserand & Balacs (1995, p. 43) do not consider essential oils to be contraindicated in cases of hypertension or hypotension, as there is insufficient evidence to suggest that they are hazardous. They list certain constituents as being hypotensors: linalol, citronellol, nerol, geraniol, terpineol and cineole (in descending order of effectiveness).

Certain oils are known to trigger epileptic fits and should be avoided in women with epilepsy and in those with fulminating pre-eclampsia. Interactions with pharmaceutical drugs should also be considered, although those listed by Tisserand & Balacs (1995, p. 43) are generally essential oils not normally used for pregnancy and childbearing (see also Chapter 4).

Nutmeg is contraindicated in mothers receiving pethidine, and care should be taken when using essential oils in conjunction with certain tranquillizers, anticonvulsants and antihistamines – although it is probably wise to check biosynthetic pathways and drug interactions for any woman before using essential oils. This will not usually pose a problem for midwives as most of the women for whom they care are fit and healthy and unlikely to be receiving medication; those already under medical supervision will possibly not be suitable for the administration of essential oils. However, practitioners working independently should seek the relevant expert advice if they are unsure about possible interactions of essential oils with existing medication. Geranium is reputed to have an anticoagulant effect and is therefore contraindicated in women receiving warfarin; aromatherapy for these women and those with cardiac disease should be administered only after full consultation between the consultants and the midwife, who should be a fully trained and experienced therapist. It is worth noting, however, that some oils stimulate the heart and should be used with caution in all women during pregnancy and the puerperium when massive cardiovascular adaptations are taking place. These include black pepper, caraway, hyssop, nutmeg and thyme.

Rubefacient (warming) oils would be unsuitable for pyrexial women, as would those that increase perspiration. These include basil, black pepper, cajeput, camomile, eucalyptus, fennel, garlic, ginger, hyssop, juniper, lavender, melissa, myrrh, peppermint, rosemary and tea tree, although tea tree is valuable in cases where the pyrexia is due to infection.

Most essential oils are excreted via the kidneys, but certain oils increase diuresis and can be helpful for fluid retention or postpartum oedema. They are contraindicated, however, after severe blood loss. Essential oils in this category include benzoin, black pepper, camomile, carrot seed, cedarwood, cypress, eucalyptus, fennel, garlic, geranium, hyssop, juniper, lavender, lemon, parsley, patchouli, rose, rosemary, sage and sandalwood. Independent aromatherapists who are not midwives should seek the advice of the conventional maternity care team regarding the use of massage of the abdomen following postpartum haemorrhage. Products retained in utero may cause abdominal discomfort during massage, or the massage may itself, in a few cases, precipitate further haemorrhage.

These examples demonstrate the importance of a thorough understanding of both the physiology of the childbearing phase and the potential effects of essential oils on both the mother and the fetus. Oils that can be used to treat specific conditions are discussed more fully in Chapter 7.

In labour the same criteria for selection of oils as in pregnancy should be considered. Some of those that are considered abortifacient can be used with care, but they would be contraindicated in women at risk of haemorrhage. Postnatally it is necessary to be aware of the history of pregnancy and labour, and then to review the desirable and unacceptable effects of the oils to be used. Obviously many essential oils that were contraindicated in pregnancy may now be used, although those that induce uterine bleeding should be administered with caution until the lochia have subsided. For the neonate only very low dilutions (i.e. 0.5–1%) of gentle essential oils should be used, and it is advised that this is restricted to camomile or mandarin. In many instances simple massage with a base oil can be effective and is certainly safer if there is any doubt about individual essential oils. The fragility of the skin in preterm neonates does, however, mean that any massage should be performed extremely gently.

Health and safety issues

There are several issues that need to be taken into account when using essential oils, especially for pregnant and childbearing women, and most particularly when care is provided in institutional settings such as the maternity unit. Some of the considerations apply to the method of administration of the essential oils and are dealt with in Chapter 6. This section is specifically concerned with health and safety from a legal perspective and focuses on the fact that essential oils are chemical substances that could potentially be hazardous to health.

Essential oils are subject to the regulations pertaining to Control of Substances Hazardous to Health 1994 (COSHH) and Chemical Hazard Information and Packaging for Supply 1994 (CHIPS), as well as aspects of the Health and Safety at Work Act. It is necessary to undertake a risk assessment on all essential oils in use, in order to identify possible adverse effects, not only on the clients to whom they are administered, but also on the therapists, their colleagues and employers and any other people who may be exposed to the oils, e.g. visitors in the maternity unit.

Safety data sheets are available for all chemical substances and should state safety information in relation to toxicological effects, storage, handling, spillage, first aid, fire, personal protective equipment, where appropriate, and other relevant advice. It is possible to obtain safety data sheets for all essential oils from the suppliers, although even those that detail the chemical components of the oils may be inadequate for the risk assessment. Essential oils should be classified in categories ranging from relatively harmless through to extremely toxic. The CHIPS regulations require chemical containers to be labelled adequately with the supplier's name and address and their appropriate chemical danger category as well as other relevant information. Fowler & Wall (1997) express concern at the confusion that exists in aromatherapy, even among the most renowned authorities, about the properties, precautions and contraindications of different oils; this is echoed by Vickers (1997). This is particularly pertinent to caring for pregnant and childbearing women, and for the assessment of risk to pregnant workers.

Fowler & Wall (1998) suggest that, in order to undertake a risk assessment of the essential oils in use, therapists should consider the following issues (maternity-specific points have been added by this author):

◆ A record should be made of all essential oils in use with research-based information on their properties, potential side-effects, precautions and contraindications, from which a decision can be made as to whether the oil is relatively harmless or not.

◆ The volatility of essential oils means that they all carry a fire risk and this should be taken into account, especially in relation to vaporization of oils. All electrical vaporizers used in institutional settings must be checked by a qualified and experienced electrician before use and regularly thereafter.

◆ Siting of aromatherapy treatment is important in an institutional setting since individuals other than the client may inhale the vapours; having a designated room available may reduce the risk. Environmental fragrancing is inappropriate in a maternity unit but care should be taken when treatments are provided for women in traditional 'Nightingale' style wards. Exposure of medical and midwifery staff to certain essential oils, especially those known to be sedative, could potentially adversely affect clinical judgement.

◆ Ventilation of the room must be adequate, although specialized ducting is probably unnecessary. Where a room is to be used for other clients afterwards windows and doors should be left open to ensure a through draft.

◆ Hygiene facilities should be provided for therapists, clients and others.

◆ Disposal of essential oil materials and containers must be considered – possibly in sealed metal containers because of their flammability.

◆ 'Safer' essential oils could be substitued for those thought to be too toxic or potentially harmful.

◆ Protective gloves may be desirable for the therapist, at least during pouring and blending of essential oils, even if not for administering the actual treatment.

◆ All essential oils should be stored appropriately in a locked cupboard or refrigerator, according to the storage requirements for each oil.

Conclusion   It is vital that the possible dangers of essential oils are recognized. The lack of adequate research findings in relation to pregnancy and childbearing means that both midwives and aromatherapists currently have limited knowledge on which to base their practice. Great caution should be exercised when caring for pregnant women who wish to receive aromatherapy. It is not the intention of the author to dissuade practitioners from using essential oils for pregnant clients, but rather to highlight the effects that the chemistry or pharmacological actions may have upon them. Pregnant women who request information about using essential oils at this time should be advised to purchase only good-quality products and to use dilutions of 1–2%, preferably with reference to an appropriately qualified practitioner as to the safest and most therapeutically valuable oils.

This author would strongly advise midwives and aromatherapists treating pregnant women to use only the lowest doses necessary to achieve the desired results, avoiding prolonged administration of any one oil (or those with similar levels of the same constituents), and to refrain from using most essential oils until the second trimester. Practitioners must be able to justify their choice of essential oils and must know thoroughly the actions, contraindications and side-effects of the oils that they administer. While these principles apply to the use of aromatherapy for all clients, special attention must be paid to the fact that two human beings are being treated during pregnancy.

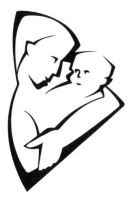

Chapter 6 # Administration of Essential Oils

Essential oils can be administered in many ways: via the skin or mucous membranes through massage, baths, compresses, douches or enemas, or via the respiratory tract as inhalations or in vaporizers. Essential oils may also be given orally to be absorbed through the gastrointestinal tract, but should be prescribed only by very experienced or medically qualified aromatherapists; this route of administration is not considered here.

The choice of method may depend on several factors. First, the condition being treated may dictate the route of administration; for example a cough or a cold is best treated with inhalations so that the essential oils act directly on the respiratory tract. On the other hand, women seeking aromatherapy for relief of stress would benefit most from a massage; many research trials are concerned with deciding whether the relaxation obtained is a result of the chemical constituents of the essential oils or of the massage itself.

Second, factors such as time may play a part. Where midwives are using aromatherapy in their practice, this might lead to the decision to use essential oils in the bath or bidet rather than giving a massage, which requires a longer period of undisturbed time than may be available. However, when more or less continuous one-to-one care is given, as in the delivery suite, massage can be appropriate for relieving pain and helping to relax the mother. It is unlikely that members of the conventional maternity services will be in a position to offer full body massage, except in isolated cases, and women wishing to receive regular antenatal aromatherapy should be advised to consult an independent aromatherapist with particular expertise in caring for pregnant women.

Third, and perhaps most important, the preference of the client for a particular method must be taken into account. Some women dislike being touched, especially during labour, and this must be respected by offering alternative ways of receiving essential oils; others prefer showering to bathing so that adding essential oils to the bathwater is not feasible.

Fourth, professional accountability of the practitioner must be taken into account, including ethicolegal, health and safety and educational issues. Practice must, wherever possible, be based on contemporary evidence regarding its safety and effectiveness (see also Chapter 1).

Application through the skin: massage

The application of an essential oil blend via the skin is enhanced when given via massage, which in itself can be mentally and physically relaxing, yet revitalizing. Massage also helps to stimulate circulatory and excretory processes (urinary, intestinal, lymphatic and integumentary), relaxes and tones muscles, and assists the individual quite literally to 'get in touch' with herself.

There are many types of massage, which are often used in conjunction with one another. The commonest types used in aromatherapy involve a combination of Swedish soft-tissue massage, deeper lymphatic and neuromuscular massage, shiatsu and reflexology. The specific system of therapeutic touch (TT), a system of care devised by an American nursing professor, Delores Krieger, is actually a misnomer as it does not involve physical touching of the skin but instead concentrates on massaging the aura and is not dealt with in this book. Where the term 'therapeutic touch' is used it refers simply to the therapeutic effects that physical touch (massage) can have on individuals.

In this book, with the emphasis on the use of essential oils, it is not the intention to teach the reader *how* to perform massage. Basic principles are discussed and some suggestions for the application of manual techniques to maternity care are made, but it is left to the practitioner to pursue the acquisition of specific skills elsewhere. Massage is, in any case, mostly intuitive: massage cannot be learnt from a book and there are many excellent courses (and more detailed course texts) available (see Further reading and Appendix 3: Useful Addresses). Readers are referred also to the excellent video 'A Practical Guide to Childbirth Massage Techniques' produced by Talking Pictures (1999).

Swedish soft-tissue massage   Swedish massage consists of several types of movement: stroking (effleurage), a deep thumb massage called petrissage, kneading and percussion movements.

Effleurage   Effleurage is a slow flowing movement in which the body is stroked by the whole hand, which changes shape to fit the contours of the body. Movements are normally directed towards the heart to stimulate circulation and lymphatic drainage, although effleurage at the end of a massage tends to encourage removal of tension from the body by outwards movements along the limbs and up the head. Effleurage may be fairly light for work on the nervous system and for helping to relax the woman emotionally, although not so light as to cause tickling sensations. It may also be a deeper movement for work on specific tense muscles and to improve blood flow.

Effleurage is used to link other movements and can be performed on any part of the body; if in doubt about what to do in a massage, effleurage will enhance a woman's sense of relaxation and wellbeing. The tendency of the novice masseuse to work too lightly will be overcome with increasing confidence, and practitioners will come to know the appropriate pressure to use. For example, the back and limbs often respond to deep firm pressure, whereas the pregnant or labouring woman may want featherlight effleurage in a clockwise circular movement over the abdomen. She can be shown how to do this herself during pregnancy and many women report the calming of a very active fetus when they have done so. Similarly, effleurage of the face will need a much lighter touch, as will effleurage of babies – in this latter case pressure will instinctively be adjusted by the practitioner in much the same way as a midwife or paediatrician adapts the pressure of cardiopulmonary resuscitation for adults or babies.

Effleurage can be performed with one hand or both, either together or alternately; in straight flowing lines following the contours of the body or in circles of varying sizes. Different pressures and speeds, perhaps even pausing and holding occasionally, will provide variety in the massage and prevent boredom in both the recipient and the therapist.

Petrissage   Petrissage involves deeper work with the thumbs on more precise areas of the body and may be effective in reducing motor neuron excitability (Goldberg et al 1992, Morelli et al 1990, Sullivan et al 1991). Soft tissues, primarily muscles, are compressed, either against underlying bone or against themselves, and the movements may be in the form of kneading, wringing, rolling or shaking manipulations.

Kneading   Kneading is a circular, squeezing movement performed with the whole hand, using the fingers and thumbs to pick up fleshy parts of the body or to compress the tissues against the underlying structures. The movement may be performed with the whole hand, the palm, the fingers, or the tips of the fingers and thumbs. Kneading is a very useful technique for dealing with aching, tense muscles as it stimulates the local circulation and disperses any lactic acid that may have built up in the muscles. Spontaneous massage of the shoulders is a kneading movement of the flesh over the trapezius muscle.

Occasionally the tissues of the body are compressed using a 'picking up' technique to lift, squeeze and release them. In a wringing movement, the tissues are compressed, lifted then pulled and pushed by alternate hands, while another technique involves rolling the skin and, in some instances, the underlying muscles.

Percussion movements   Percussion movements (sometimes called tapotement) include cupping and hacking, which are perhaps the two movements most readily associated with Swedish massage. They involve brisk, bouncy movements on fleshy parts of the body to improve circulation and re-energize the recipient. Hacking is done with the distal edges of the hands, which bounce alternately at right angles to the client's body, and has been shown to improve blood flow in skeletal muscles (Hovind & Nielson 1974).

Cupping movements are performed with the therapist's palms directed downwards and slightly arched; this is the action carried out by physiotherapists to stimulate chest drainage. Both cupping and hacking should be followed by effleurage to soothe and calm; in some cases these movements are omitted altogether as they may disturb the deep relaxation, particularly when the aim of the massage is to induce sleep.

Benefits of massage   Generally massage has been found to reduce heart and respiratory rates and blood pressure (Barr & Taslitz 1970; see also Box 6.1), although a trial involving cardiothoracic patients did not demonstrate significant cardiovascular changes (Bauer & Dracup 1987). Cardiovascular instability was put forward as a possible contraindication to massage in critically ill patients (Hill 1993) (see Box 6.2 for contraindications). Massage does, however, increase the individual's sense of wellbeing (Farrow 1990, Field et al 1993, Fraser & Kerr 1993, McKechnie et al 1983, Sims 1986) and reduce pain perception (Day et al 1987, Ferrell-Torry & Glick 1993, Ginsberg & Famaey 1987, Kaada & Torsteinbo 1989; see Box 6.1). Women who receive touch during labour, particularly in the transition phase, have been shown to be more relaxed, to have lower blood pressures, to experience less pain and to feel more satisfied post-delivery than control subjects who were not touched (Birch 1986, Hedstrom & Newton 1986, Le May 1986). Perception of pain can be adversely or positively affected by a woman's mental state, so that fear and anxiety will exacerbate the pain, while nurturing care will assist in reducing it. This may be the result of the release of pituitary endorphins, which facilitate a sense of wellbeing; the possible interruption of transmission of pain impulses to the brain; and the stimulation of inhibitory interneurons in the spinal cord that lessen pain perception.

Box 6.1   Benefits of massage

Physical	Psychological
Muscle relaxation	Mental relaxation
Sudorific	Revitalizing
Lowers blood pressure	Releases emotions
Stimulates circulation	Facilitates communication
Increases diuresis	Aids sleep
Stimulates lymphatic drainage	Time for oneself
Reduces oedema	
Pain relieving	

Box 6.2   Contraindications and precautions of massage

General
Infection, contagious disease, pyrexia
Skin problems – inflammation, open wounds, burns, severe bruising
Varicosities – avoid direct pressure
Thrombophlebitis or phlebothrombosis
Sciatica – take care around this area
Recent fractures, scars – avoid direct pressure
Carcinoma – avoid direct massage over relevant area
Recent immunizations – avoid direct pressure
Immediately after ingestion of heavy meal or alcohol
Hypotension – monitor blood pressure closely
Preference of client

Pregnancy: specific
Sacral and suprapubic massage during first trimester
Deep massage of calves if history of thrombosis
Brisk heel massage – reflexology zone for pelvic area
Shiatsu points contraindicated in pregnancy (see Fig. 6.1)
Hypotension or fainting episodes – monitor blood pressure closely
Abdominal massage if history of antepartum haemorrhage
Uncertainty of midwife – if in doubt, refrain
Preference of client

It is also possible that various blood changes may occur as a result of massage, including an increase in the levels of creatinine kinase, lactate dehydrogenase, growth hormone and adrenocorticotrophic hormone (Arkko et al 1983), together with a decrease in blood and plasma viscosity, haematocrit (Ernst et al 1987) and, 24 hours after the massage, haemoglobin (Arkko et al 1983).

Shiatsu   Shiatsu techniques are often incorporated into aromatherapy massage and are thought to rebalance energy along the meridians (energy flow lines) throughout the body. Although it was traditionally believed that meridians were metaphorical, work has demonstrated their physical existence, as shown by electrical energy tests and radio-opaque dye tests (Bensoussan 1991).

Expert shiatsu practitioners carry out full body massage by working along each meridian of the body, but in aromatherapy only a few points are used. It would be appropriate and acceptable to incorporate shiatsu to a few specified acupuncture points for pregnant, labouring and newly delivered mothers, but it is equally important to be fully cognizant of any contraindicated points. There are certain shiatsu points that should not be stimulated during pregnancy as they may initiate preterm labour (Fig. 6.1). It is also important to ensure that the techniques are learnt properly to avoid any potential complications. *The Lancet* of February 1993 carried a report of a woman who developed herpes zoster lesions 3 days after receiving what appeared to be an overvigorous shiatsu massage. The authors

Fig. 6.1. Shiatsu points contraindicated in pregnancy.

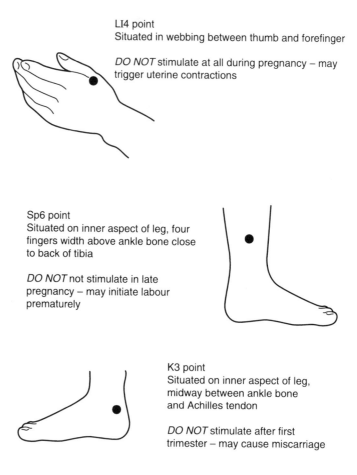

LI4 point
Situated in webbing between thumb and forefinger

DO NOT stimulate at all during pregnancy – may trigger uterine contractions

Sp6 point
Situated on inner aspect of leg, four fingers width above ankle bone close to back of tibia

DO NOT not stimulate in late pregnancy – may initiate labour prematurely

K3 point
Situated on inner aspect of leg, midway between ankle bone and Achilles tendon

DO NOT stimulate after first trimester – may cause miscarriage

surmise that nerve root damage may have occurred, either during the massage or as a result of tissue inflammation (Mumm et al 1993).

Finger pressure is applied slowly and rhythmically, never abruptly or forcefully. This slow work enables the tissue and organs of the body to respond to the treatment and prevents overstimulation of the points, which could lead to excess toxins being released, causing the mother to feel ill. For obvious reasons it is wise to avoid areas where the skin is irritated, burnt or recently scarred, and acupressure points situated over lymph glands should be touched only very lightly to avoid pain and discomfort.

Reflexology   Reflexology is a manual treatment in which the feet represent a map of the body, so that by working on specific parts of the feet other areas of the body can be treated. Although it is not known how reflexology works, the Eastern theory is that it involves similar principles to acupressure: by working on the meridians in the feet treatment is directed to related zones in the body. The Western theory relates to the nervous system, with manipulation of the nerve endings in the feet influencing other parts of the body. Although reflexology is not a standard element of aromatherapy massage, and does not normally involve the use of oils, it can occasionally serve as an alternative or complement to other manual therapies used in massage (see also Tiran & Mack 2000). However, it must also be recognized that reflexology or reflex zone therapy is potentially harmful if misused, either through ignorance or intention. A thorough understanding of the physiology of childbearing is necessary before a practitioner commences reflexology on a pregnant or labouring woman; this applies equally to shiatsu (see Chapter 1).

Baby massage Massage of the neonate, either by mothers or professionals, has become extremely popular recently as it is recognized that touch can be so soothing. There are many reports of midwives, health visitors and therapists establishing classes at which parents can learn and become confident in massaging their infants (Adamson 1996a, Bowers-Clarke 1993, Chaplin 1996, Curran 1996, Isherwood 1994, Lim 1996, Mason 1996), although it must be stressed that professionals should be adequately trained to offer this service. A Certified Infant Massage Instructors Course is now available in the UK, under the auspices of the International Association of Infant Massage (Adamson 1996b).

The benefits of regular baby massage, especially in preterm infants, have been shown to be an enhanced parent–infant relationship (Ineson 1995, Walker 1995, White-Traut & Nelson 1988), maintenance of body temperature (Johanson et al 1992), enhanced maturation and growth (Field et al 1986, Kuhn et al 1991) and improved prognosis for intellectual development (Adamson-Macedo et al 1993). This is in direct contrast to the hitherto conventional policies of 'minimal handling' of preterm babies; different types of handling, whether nurturing or functional, produce different responses (Appleton 1997), and Adamson-Macedo et al's study (1997) seems to indicate that systematic gentle/light stroking is not detrimental to oxygen saturation levels. This TAC-TIC therapy (Touching And Caressing, Tender In Caring) has previously been advocated (Adamson-Macedo et al 1993, 1994a, 1994b, de Roiste & Bushnell 1995, de Roiste et al 1995).

For the parents, physical contact with the baby will increase their confidence in general handling and can indirectly help to relax them – fretful babies lead to distressed mothers and this is in turn transmitted back to the baby so that the whole episode becomes a vicious circle. Teaching parents to massage their baby is one of the easiest and most pleasant means of achieving a good family relationship and should be promoted from birth. Parents can be encouraged to follow the bath time with a few valuable minutes spent stroking the baby, perhaps as they apply baby lotion, talcum powder or oil.

After feeding, the mother could maintain contact with her baby, just gently stroking the back and head, rather than concentrating on the outmoded 'winding', which is still suggested on occasions. If any investigations such as phenylkentonuria or serum bilirubin tests are required, the mother could sit with the infant on her knee and massage accessible areas of the body, or simply hold the baby's hand. Baby massage classes provide an opportunity for parents not only to develop further their relationship with their child, but also offer valuable access to a midwife or health visitor, who may achieve more in less time than seeing mothers individually at routine child health clinics. Therapists who are not midwives or health visitors may establish infant massage classes, which also provide a valuable forum for social interaction for the mothers.

Even when a neonate is seriously ill, the parents could insert a hand into the incubator and maintain contact by stroking the baby's head, hand or leg. This does not have to be intrusive and interfere with any necessary technology, but can facilitate for the parents a sense of belonging and of being involved in the care of their baby. Initially it will require the midwives or neonatal nurses to suggest the various ways of touching the baby, but will probably occur spontaneously if parents observe the staff also enjoying regular contact with the child. This will serve as a form of 'permission giving' to parents who may feel afraid to touch the baby – a baby who seems to belong more to the staff than themselves. Midwives and neonatal nurses should constantly be considering ways in which they can demonstrate the benefits of touch, and set an example to the parents, particularly in view of research findings that suggest that tactile stimulation of seriously ill neonates can have positive effects on sympathetic and adrenocortical function (Acolet et al 1993, Kuhn et al 1991), temperature maintenance (Johanson et al 1992) heart rate and oxygen saturation (Harrison et al 1990, Helders et al 1988).

Views on whether preterm infants should be touched or left undisturbed have changed radically in the past few years, but there may be occasions when massage is contraindicated. These include hyperpyrexial infants, in whom the vasodilatory effects of massage could severely compromise the condition; babies whose cerebral condition is so unstable that tactile communication may initiate a fit; those with major cardiac conditions; and infected neonates. Common sense on the part of the staff will help them to decide whether an individual baby seems well enough to receive some form of massage or touch therapy.

Application through the skin: in water

Essential oils can be administered in the bathwater providing a pleasant smelling and relaxing experience. The oils should be diluted to the required dosage (see 'The art of blending essential oils' below) and should not be dropped into the water neat. This is because oil will float on the surface of the water; if the neat oil then comes in contact with the skin it may cause irritation. Therefore, the oils can be blended with either the normal base oil or in another fluid that facilitates dispersion, such as full cream milk, very mild shampoo or even vodka (although this does seem rather a waste of vodka!).

If an aromatic bath is considered appropriate, the essential oils should be added to the water after the bath is filled, and dispersed thoroughly; if the oils are added while the hot tap is running, the steam will cause the volatile oils to evaporate. Alternatively, sprigs of fresh herbs can be hung under the stream of water as it fills the bath.

The temperature and depth of the water will depend on the purpose for which the bath is being taken. If the object is to aid relaxation and induce sleep, a deep but tepid bath is best; to invigorate, a short, hot shallower bath can be effective – but very hot water can be debilitating if the bath is prolonged. Pregnant women should be discouraged from very hot baths in any case, as their temperature is already raised as a result of increased blood volume.

For a general de-stressing soak it is pleasant to be able to submerge under deep water, although this may not always be practical. Mothers wishing to labour in the bath may have essential oils added if the membranes are intact, but once ruptured the water should be changed. If delivery takes place in the bath no essential oils should be used; this is to avoid the risk to the baby's eyes of coming in contact with the oils. Garland (2000, p. 233) states that in her unit no other means of analgesia is used when women labour in the bath, as the water itself is intended as a pain reliever, although Lichy & Herzberg (1993, p. 119) suggest that the addition of 'a few drops' of essential oil to the bathwater can be helpful. This author advocates a cautious approach to the use of essential oils during water birth, in line with Garland's comments.

Where localized wounds such as Caesarean section or episiotomy are to be bathed, the water must obviously be high enough to cover the afflicted area, although a bidet could also be used for perineal bathing. Foot baths are a practical method of providing aromatherapy as they enable the mother to receive essential oils systemically yet use little water and do not require much supervision. One often-quoted anecdote, which indicates how quickly essential oils are transported around the body, is that of a test in which essential oil of garlic was applied to the subject's feet, and within 20 minutes the odour was detectable on his breath.

Compresses Compresses can be made by soaking a cloth (a sanitary towel is especially good) in the water to which the essential oils have previously been added; the excess is squeezed out and the compress applied to the affected area. This is a particularly effective and efficient method during labour when the mother may wish to receive aromatherapy in a form other than massage and yet feels unable to climb in and out of a bath, or if bathrooms in the maternity unit are all in use. Compresses applied to the suprapubic and sacral areas during the first stage using oils such as clary sage can be comforting and analgesic, and in the second and third stages lavender and/or jasmine may enhance uterine action.

Vulval washes   Vulval washes may be used for infections, leucorrhoea and as a general hygiene measure; tea tree-soaked tampons are excellent for treating vaginal thrush. Douches are recommended by many aromatherapy authorities but should be used with caution during the child-bearing period and avoided once the membranes have ruptured and in the puerperium to minimize the dangers of fluid embolism entering the circulation via the placental site.

Although it is acceptable for essential oils to be used in jacuzzis and saunas, these methods of administration are contraindicated in pregnancy. Jacuzzis should be avoided because of the risk of embolism if water enters the vagina; saunas will raise the mother's temperature to a level that could adversely affect the fetus.

Application via the respiratory tract   Inhalation of essential oils is a logical means of administration for conditions specifically affecting the respiratory tract, although, as with other applications, the effects will eventually be systemic. Where mothers are suffering from a cold, influenza, sinus congestion or postoperative chest infection, essential oils can be added to hot water and given via traditional inhalation apparatus or simply by leaning over the bowl with a towel covering the head to direct the vapours towards the nostrils. This latter method can also be used as a facial sauna in cases of acne or other skin conditions.

Various items of equipment are now available to facilitate diffusion of essential oils (Fig. 6.2). Some are decorative pots incorporating a heat source such as a night-light candle, which helps the volatile essential oils to evaporate. However, those with a naked flame contravene institutional health and safety regulations and should never be used in the maternity unit. If a mother chooses to use one in the home she should be advised about safe positioning, remembering that in labour she may inadvertently move an arm or leg and knock it over if it is too close.

Other devices for vaporizing essential oils include small porcelain rings. Two or three essential oil drops (without water) are added to the ring, which is rested on an upturned light bulb for its heat source, or essential oils can be added to a humidifier or a small bowl of water positioned on top of a radiator.

Electrical vaporizers are the most suitable for use in the maternity unit and, despite the additional cost, are safer and more durable. They are useful in the labour ward where mothers are normally in single rooms, but should be turned on intermittently; this is to prevent the aroma from becoming overpowering and to avoid 'aroma immunity'. Ten minutes of vaporization in each hour will probably be sufficient; on no account should the vaporizer be left on constantly. Mothers and independent aromatherapists accompanying women into the delivery suite must be aware of the need for a hospital electrician to check the safety of any electrical equipment brought in; it is not feasible to expect this to be accomplished during the relatively short episode of a woman's labour.

Fig. 6.2. *Equipment for vaporizing essential oils.*

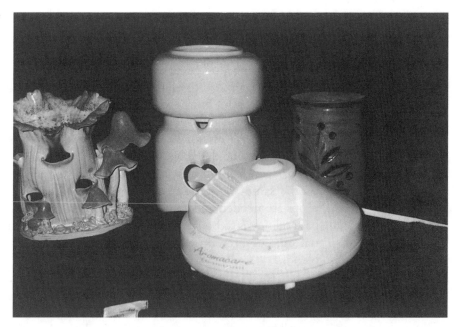

Room sprays can be made using 10 drops of a blend of essential oils in approximately 200 ml of water. Lemon essential oil makes a refreshing room deodorizer and freshener. Pot pourri can also, of course, be used, with the essential oils being added every few days.

For mothers who have difficulty in sleeping, two drops of an essential oil such as lavender or camomile, according to preference, can be put directly on to the pillow; likewise fretful babies can benefit from application of *one* drop of camomile oil on the sheet near their heads. For pregnant women with sinus congestion, two drops of tea tree or marjoram oil on a cotton handkerchief and sniffed at intervals can provide relief. In labour the nausea and vomiting experienced by many women may be relieved by putting two drops of peppermint or spearmint essential oil onto a cotton wool ball or gauze for inhalation as required.

The art of blending essential oils

The choice of essential oils to be used for a mother depends on several factors. The therapeutic requirements are obviously of prime importance, together with an acknowledgement of any contraindications to specific oils. Essential oil chemicals have both physiological and psychological effects, the latter as a result of the aromas working directly on the brain through the olfactory organ (see Chapter 4).

It is perfectly acceptable to select a single essential oil in a carrier but up to five essential oils may be blended together if this is justified, although using a single oil would assist in identifying any untoward side-effects, enabling those that adversely affect a mother to be avoided. Essential oils are known to work synergistically, however; in other words, the total effect of a blend is more than the sum of its parts, with one oil enhancing the action of another.

Dosage   The dosage of essential oils for use in pregnancy and labour should be no more than 1–2% for massage, preferably less in pregnancy; and 4% for baths. For newly delivered mothers a 2–3% blend can be used (4–6% in baths), and neonates should never receive more than a 1% blend at any time. All essential oils should be added to a base or carrier oil, and the amount calculated as follows.

For each 5 millilitres (ml) of base oil the number of drops added will be the same as the percentage blend required, e.g. for a 2% blend, two drops are needed and so on. When 1.5% blend is favoured, the amount of base oil needs to be doubled, as it is not possible to add half drops of essential oil, i.e. three drops of oil are added to 10 ml base oil to make 1.5% blend.

The total number of drops must never exceed that required when only one oil is used, so that if a 2% mix using lavender and mandarin is wanted, only one drop of each is added to 5 ml base oil. This does, however, pose a challenge to the aromatherapist, for how does she decide on the most appropriate balance of essential oils when more than one is used?

Let us consider a mother with postnatal urinary tract infection, for which the aromatherapist decided to use a 2.5% blend of bergamot and sandalwood, both of which are thought to have an affinity for the urinary tract. This would mean that to 10 ml of base oil five drops of essential oil should be added – but in what proportions? It is probable that the practitioner would chose two drops of one oil and three drops of the other; from an aromatic viewpoint it would be preferable for sandalwood to be in the greater proportion for this oil takes a while to warm up and become a noticeable aroma. (It is worth noting Watt's comments (personal communication, 1995, 1996) that it may simply be the performance of massage, irrespective of which essential oil is used, that facilitates diuresis. Similarly, many other oils are known to possess various anti-infective properties.)

In cases where several essential oils are used together, it is partly a knowledge of each oil's therapeutic properties, partly client preference and partly experience of the art of blending that dictates the selection of the proportion of oils. Essential oil molecules begin the process of evaporation as soon as they are exposed to the air and continue for varying lengths of time, according to the volatility of the oil and other factors that may accelerate the process. This degeneration causes a constantly changing chemical composition as some constituents evaporate faster than others.

Consequently the aromas alter, albeit subtly. Certainly the initial fresh aroma will eventually give way to one that is the main 'theme' of the essential oil blend. This will be followed at a later stage by a different, more persistent, odour that will endure for anything up to 8 hours.

The 'notes' system of blending   These chemical changes led to the development by a perfumer, Septimus Piesse, in the nineteenth century of a system of 'notes' to facilitate the creation of harmonious perfumes. There are now more sophisticated methods in use but the principles still apply and can be adapted for creativity in aromatherapy.

As a general rule, essential oils extracted from the tops of plants – the flowers and fruit – are the 'top' notes, providing fresh fruity aromas immediately noticeable on blending but relatively short-lived. These include the citrus essences and other distinctive sharp aromas such as lemongrass, ginger and eucalyptus.

Essential oils from the whole plant, leaves and stems, i.e. the middle part of the plant, constitute the 'middle' notes, which are often used as the main therapeutic oil of the blend. This includes most of the herbal oils. The 'base' notes are those oils extracted from the base of the plant, e.g. the roots, seed, bark and wood. They have aromas that emerge only after warming of the oil but which linger the longest; they include carrot seed, sandalwood and rosewood.

A useful comparison to help understanding of this concept of notes is to consider the drug Syntometrine®, given intramuscularly to aid placental separation. Within this drug the oxytocin component works rapidly to initiate an almost immediate uterine contraction and to force the placenta to separate from the decidua, but its action is short-lived. The work of this 'synergistic' blend of drugs is then taken over by ergometrine, which takes several minutes to have an effect but whose action is then sustained to prevent uterine relaxation and consequent haemorrhage.

Other methods of blending   Many aromatherapists use the notes system of blending to help their choice of essential oils. Another method is to blend oils that originate from the same family, for example citrus essences (Rutaceae family) or herbal oils (Labiatae family). Oils that contain the same chemical constituents marry well, such as those containing the aldehyde citronella (eucalyptus, melissa, mandarin and lemongrass), while on the other hand some chemical constituents 'compete' aromatically, making the resultant blend unacceptable.

Essential oils from the same parts of plants enhance each other, for example those from fruits or from woods. A few essential oils, such as lavender and rose, are extremely versatile and blend well with a large number of other oils, whereas others have such a distinctive aroma that their flexibility is limited, e.g. garlic.

Much of the art of blending essential oils comes from an instinctive feel for what is right – and some therapists are better at blending than others. One of the easiest ways of selecting oils is to remove the bottle tops from those being considered and waft them slowly past the nostrils of both the client and practitioner. This will give an idea of whether the oils enhance or compete with each other, but it is really only with continued practice that individuals become 'nasally tuned in' and adept at selecting oils that blend well.

Many of the main chemical constituents of essential oils have now been identified, through scientific analysis, as having specific odour classifications. There are also many less commonly found or as yet undiscovered chemicals still to be classified; a few examples are given in Table 6.1.

Table 6.1
Odour
classification
of some
chemical
constituents of
essential oils

Constituent	Odour	Essential oil
Aldehydes		
Cinnamic aldehyde	Cinnamon-like	Cinnamon
Citral	Citrus, lemon	Mandarin
Citronellal	Citrus, rose-like	Lemon
Esters		
Benzyl acetate	Floral, fruity	Ylang ylang
Bornyl acetate	Camphorous	Rosemary
Geranyl acetate	Sweet, rose-like, fruity	Lemongrass
Linalyl acetate	Light, herbal, slightly fruity	Clary sage
Neryl acetate	Sweet, rose-like, fruity	Neroli
Alcohols		
Borneol	Woody, camphorous	Rosemary
Cedrol	Faintly woody	Cypress
Citronellol	Rich, floral, rose-like	Geranium
Linalol	Floral, woody, slightly spicy	Basil
Menthol	Fresh, minty	Peppermint
Nerol	Sweet, floral, slightly seaweedy	Neroli
Ketones		
Camphor	Fresh, warm, minty	Marjoram
Fenchone	Warm, camphorous	Fennel
Menthone	Minty, slightly woody	Peppermint
Thujone	Strong, herbal, camphorous	Sage
Phenols		
Carvacrol	Tar-like, herbal, spicy	Thyme
Estragol	Sweet, herbal, aniseed-like	Fennel
Eugenol	Spicy, clove-like	Marjoram
Methyl chavicol	Similar to estragol	Basil
Safrole	Warm, spicy, woody	Nutmeg
Oxides		
1,8-Cineole	Eucalyptus-like	Eucalyptus
Monoterpenes		
Camphene	Camphorous	Juniper
Limonene	Weak citrus	Grapefruit
Myrcene	Sweet, balsamic	Black pepper
Phellandrene	Citrus, spicy, woody	Frankincense
Pinene	Woody, pine-like	Petitgrain
Sesquiterpenes		
α-Terpinene	Fresh, citrus-like	Tea tree
β-Bisabolene	Balsamic, spicy	Camomile
Sabinene	Spicy, woody, herbal	Juniper

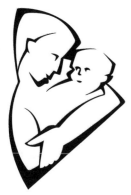

Chapter 7 **Using Essential Oils in Maternity Care**

It has been emphasized elsewhere in this book that the benefits of using essential oils for the childbearing woman and her infant must be balanced by a thorough working knowledge of the potential hazards of the substances. Aromatherapy is as safe a system of care as any other when used by appropriately trained and experienced practitioners, but in a similar way to pharmacological preparations is open either to inadvertent or intentional misuse.

However, there are many situations within maternity care when aromatherapy can be of great value, and this chapter addresses those occasions. In some instances it may be appropriate to use essential oils in conjunction with conventional care, perhaps to relieve stress; in others, aromatherapy is used as an alternative, either as essential oils or as a herbal infusion. In some cases, manual techniques including shiatsu and reflexology may be appropriate, with or without essential oils, and suggestions are made for incorporating these into the care of the mothers and babies; where other complementary therapies may be more effective, these have not been dealt with here and the reader is referred to the list of further reading for additional information.

Appetite changes

Expectant and newly delivered mothers may find that their appetite changes. This may be a reduced desire to eat, perhaps due to physiological effects such as nausea, or an increase in appetite (probably because oestrogen is an appetite stimulant), and occasionally cravings or pica, thought to be due to certain dietary deficiencies.

Essential oil of bergamot may act as an appetite regulator, making it useful for either a loss of or an increase in appetite. As far as is known, this oil is safe to use during pregnancy and could be given to the mother to add to her bath. Small amounts of bergamot are found in Earl Grey tea, although some women dislike the taste of tea in pregnancy and find the tannin exacerbates constipation.

Essential oils of marjoram, thyme and melissa are suggested as appetite stimulants by Ryman (1991, p. 233), while Valnet (1982, p. 200) also recommends, camomile, caraway coriander, hyssop, juniper, nutmeg, origanum, sage and tarragon; although these are not suitable for use in pregnancy some such as camomile may be helpful postpartum. Sage, however, is definitely contraindicated during the childbearing phase, even after delivery while lochia is being discharged, because of its tendency to induce or increase uterine bleeding, and should probably be avoided altogether in women of reproductive years unless under the control of an experienced aromatherapist. Culinary use of the relevant herbs could be an alternative means of ingesting the active ingredients.

Fresh lemon or lime juice can assist in removing a sour taste from the mouth, especially if the expectant mother has been vomiting; inhaling essential oil of lime may reduce pica or relieve excess salivation, which can sometimes be a distressing problem. Ginger and lemongrass are also thought to stimulate the appetite, although the aroma may exacerbate nausea in some women. Fennel, often quoted as an appetite stimulant, is not suitable for administration in pregnancy.

Backache Backache in pregnancy is extremely common owing to the influence of the hormones relaxin and progesterone and the consequent lumbar lordosis that occurs as compensation for the increasing abdominal growth and weight. There is often a sense of instability in the groin and hip areas and occasionally sciatica radiating down the legs. The pelvic girdle reacts to the influence of hormones enabling it to stretch slightly to facilitate delivery. These hormonal and structural changes can have long-term effects on the mother for up to a year following delivery.

Aromatherapy can be useful in easing backache but care must be taken with sacral massage during pregnancy owing to the nerve plexus and location of acupuncture points which, if overstimulated, could trigger uterine contractions and result in preterm labour. It is unlikely that the mother will be able to lie prone for very long to receive back massage; in the first trimester pressure on the breasts and the abdominal area over the bladder may be too uncomfortable and may accentuate the lumbar curve; in late pregnancy the abdomen may be too large even to contemplate this position, although special support cushions are available to facilitate this.

If the mother is able to lie on her front, caution should be exercised when helping her to sit up afterwards. The mother should first roll onto her side, then push herself up to a sitting position, pause and then slowly stand. This will reduce the effects of postural hypotension often experienced in pregnancy, and avoid undue tension on the muscles and ligaments of the back caused by moving directly from a horizontal to an upright position.

Simple massage with base oil may be sufficient to ease backache but can be enhanced by the use of some essential oils, although those most appro-

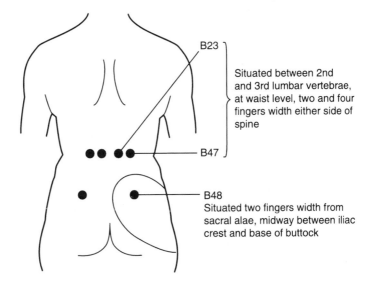

Fig. 7.1. *Shiatsu points to relieve backache.*

B23

Situated between 2nd and 3rd lumbar vertebrae, at waist level, two and four fingers width either side of spine

B47

B48
Situated two fingers width from sacral alae, midway between iliac crest and base of buttock

priate for dealing with muscular pains are contraindicated in early pregnancy: lavender, marjoram and rosemary. These can be used in labour, however, and may facilitate uterine action when an occipito-posterior position of the fetus is the cause of lumbosacral pain. (Rosemary should not be used if the mother is hypertensive.) Clary sage may also be helpful where there is an occipito-posterior position, as it will act as an overall analgesic and assist in relaxing the mother.

Black pepper in small doses, perhaps combined with a relaxing oil such as mandarin, neroli or petitgrain, will be warming and can relieve acute pain. Alternatively a warm bath to which has been added a few drops of a de-stressing oil may be sufficient.

Pressure applied to the shiatsu points may be effective in relieving symptoms; sciatica and lumbosacral pain can be eased by pressure to the B23, B47 and B48 points (Fig. 7.1), although these points might be quite tender to touch at first.

Reflexology to the foot zones for the spine can also help and a full reflexology treatment may relax the mother sufficiently to work indirectly on the pain. It must be stressed, however, that these suggestions will not treat the cause, and any mother who suffers perpetual backache during pregnancy or postnatally should be referred to an osteopath or chiropractor.

Bacterial infections

Some women may be prone to bacterial infections such as asymptomatic bacteruria or vaginal infection (see also section on Vaginal infections, p. 114). Essential oils really come into their own here, for virtually all, if not every, essential oil has some anti-infective properties, especially against bacteria.

Tea tree oil and other variants of the Mrytaceae family appear to be the most effective; as far back as 1960 Feinblatt recommended cajeput-type oil to treat boils, while Walsh & Wagstaff (1987) used *Melaleuca alternifolia* (tea tree) to inhibit the growth of oral pathogens including varieties of Streptococcus, Bacteroides and Actinomyces. In Bassett et al's work (1990) tea tree was found to work more slowly than benzoyl peroxide, the conventional treatment of choice for acne, but patients reported fewer side-effects, and Raman et al's 1995 study also supported the use of tea tree oil to treat acne. *Staphylococcus aureus* was successfully inhibited with tea tree (Carson et al 1995). However, there are reports of skin irritancy from dermal application of tea tree (Southwell et al 1997).

Various eucalyptus strains have also been found to be effective against bacterial growth (Gundidza et al 1993, Hajji & Fkih-Tetouani 1993, Hmamouch et al 1990, Piccaglia et al 1993, Zakarya et al 1993). Lavandino (a combination of *Lavandula angustifolia* and *L. latifolia*) appears to have antibacterial effects against certain non-tubercular mycobacteria, possibly due to the interaction of the essential oil with the high lipid content of the mycobacterial cell wall (Gabbrielli et al 1988). Lemongrass, together with phenoxyethanol, inhibited *Escherichia coli* and *Staphylococcus aureus*, but not *Pseudomonas aeruginosa* (Onawunmi 1988); Ogunlana et al (1987), Alam et al (1994) and Pattnaik et al (1995) replicated these findings. Orafidiya (1993) pointed out, however, that lemongrass autoxidizes during storage, particularly when exposed to air and heat, and becomes less effective in killing bacteria. Sage was shown to be effective against a range of organisms (Jalsenjak et al 1987), but should be avoided in childbearing women until further evidence is available regarding its safety. Marjoram has both antibacterial and antifungal actions (Deans & Svoboda 1990), as do thyme, clove and basil oils (Ramanoelina et al 1987); thyme has also been used as an antibacterial agent in dentistry (Meeker & Linke 1988). One strain of basil oil, *Ocimum gratissimum*, has recently been found to be more effective against several bacteria than a range of conventional antibiotics, although *Ocimum basilicum* was shown only to be moderately antimicrobial (Ndounga & Ouamba 1997), with the active constituent thought to be thymol.

Gram-positive and Gram-negative bacteria were affected by juniper berry oil (Mishra & Chauhan 1984, Stassi 1996), some Artemesia species (Mehrotra et al 1993), tagetes (marigold) (Garg & Dengre 1986), frankincense (Abdel Wahab et al 1987), rosemary (Domokos et al 1997), carrot (Kilibarda et al 1996), angelica, geranium and cinnamon, among others (Deans & Ritchie 1987). Research in 1967 by Subba et al appeared to indicate that the citrus oils were less effective as anti-infective agents, a supposition that does not seem to have been disputed by more recent trials. Out of 17 bacteria tested, only *Pseudomonas aeruginosa* was found to be resistant to Santolina (Sacchetti et al 1995), suggesting that it, too, might be a useful antibacterial.

This may seem to be an overwhelming array of essential oils suitable for treating bacterial infections, but within maternity care the safest and most appropriate oils are probably tea tree, lavender, eucalyptus and lemongrass. These can be administered as inhalations following Caesarean section or other operative procedure where respiratory tract infection is threatened, or in the bath to prevent perineal or abdominal wound infection. In cases of urinary tract infection a compress of warm water and essential oils can be pressed against the suprapubic and sacral areas. Vaginal infections may be treated, with care, by inserting a tampon soaked in essential oil diluted in water or by gently swabbing the area with the solution.

Blood pressure

In early pregnancy maternal blood pressure falls slightly due to the action of progesterone in dilating the blood vessels. This is despite a 50% rise in cardiac output and a 40% rise in plasma volume, although these increases result in a subsequent rise in blood pressure to near-normal levels at term. During the first trimester the woman may be prone to dizziness and fainting possibly associated with postural hypotension and with nausea, and this should be taken into account when administering essential oils.

Women with a certain predisposition may develop pregnancy-induced hypertension as a result of increased weight, hormonal effects and abnormal pathology. In severe cases these women may go on to develop pre-eclampsia with the risk of eclamptic fits which are potentially fatal to mother and baby. *It is the opinion of this author that essential oils to treat severe pre-eclampsia should only be administered by midwifery- or medically qualified aromatherapists who are alert to the signs and symptoms of impending eclampsia and who are in a position to deal with it, should it occur. It is not appropriate for aromatherapists who are not adequately qualified to treat these seriously ill women.*

If a pregnant woman's blood pressure is raised, any aromatherapy treatment offered must be with the knowledge and approval of the obstetrician because of the risk of interaction with hypotensive drugs and the dangers of eclampsia. It may be, however, that the consultant is willing to try aromatherapy treatment for the mother, and there are reported cases of successful treatment of gestational hypertension using oils such as rosewood (McArdle 1992). Rosewood was also used by Waymouth (1992) for essential hypertension.

Essential oils that have been found to lower blood pressure include many that are not to be used during pregnancy such as celery, clary sage, lavender (although lavender could be used in the third trimester and both lavender and clary sage may be used in labour), marjoram and melissa. Lemon, mandarin, neroli and ylang ylang can be used safely and, combined with massage, may have the desired effect. Garlic is also a hypotensor and the mother could be advised to eat plenty of whole cloves of garlic in her diet. (Using them whole in cooking increases the amount of therapeutic ingredient but does not seem to overpower the flavour or leave an aftertaste or breath odour.) Garlic oil has been shown to reduce blood pressure (Cooperative Group for the Essential Oil of Garlic 1986) and an experiment on rats (El Tahir et al 1993a) seemed to indicate that essential oil of *Nigella sativa* may be a centrally acting hypotensor.

If the hypertension is thought to be exacerbated by stress and tension, any of the safe anti-anxiety oils could be used with massage to help relax the mother, while simple massage with a base oil could be carried out by the partner. Other manual techniques could be employed to ease associated symptoms such as nausea and vomiting, headaches and ankle oedema, while abdominal massage may calm the fetus.

It is obvious that, while the above-mentioned essential oils can be used therapeutically in cases where the blood pressure needs to be reduced, these same oils would be contraindicated in women with existing low blood pressure. This would apply to all the oils, with the exception of mandarin, lemon and garlic, during the second trimester of pregnancy when there is a physiological lowering of the blood pressure, and also during labour if the mother is receiving epidural anaesthesia, when the bupivacaine or other drugs used may artificially lower the blood pressure.

Conversely there are essential oils that raise the blood pressure and could theoretically be of use in women whose blood pressure is excessively low. These oils are normally contraindicated during pregnancy as they are emmenagogic – hyssop, sage, thyme and rosemary – but it may be appropriate to use rosemary with caution near term and in labour.

If a mother suffers from postural hypotension it may be possible to teach her a shiatsu first-aid technique, applying pressure to the K1 point on the centre of the foot where the ball of the foot joins the arch (Fig. 7.2).

On the third day after delivery Sandra was very tearful, mainly due to the fact that her ankles and feet had swollen to such an extent that the skin was excessively tight; she was constipated, and felt tired and depressed. Her blood pressure had been raised antenatally and returned to normal after the birth, but her distress seemed to be the cause of it increasing again.

On entering the room the aromatherapist was confronted by Sandra in floods of tears, but after administering Bach Rescue

Fig. 7.2.   K1 shiatsu first-aid point for postural hypotension.

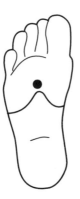

K1 point – situated on soles of feet, at base of the ball, midway between the two pads of the feet

Remedy and gently talking to Sandra she calmed down sufficiently to agree to a foot massage.

The aromatherapist used a combination of ylang ylang (to relax the mother and decrease the blood pressure), jasmine (good for postnatal depression and 'blues'), mandarin (refreshing and calming) and cypress (to reduce the oedema), and commenced firm bimanual upwards massage of the feet, ankles and lower legs. Within 5 min one foot was significantly improved, the skin felt looser and more comfortable, and Sandra was beginning to relax. Once the oedema had been dealt with, the therapist was able to incorporate reflexology to the arches of the feet, the zones for the gastrointestinal tract, to treat the constipation, and then repeat the treatment on the other foot. By the end of the 20-min session, Sandra's feet looked almost normal, she felt soporific and calm, and her diastolic blood pressure had reduced to normal limits. The next day she reported a successful bowel action, she felt much more relaxed and was normotensive once again.

Breast care

The breasts become very active during pregnancy in preparation for breastfeeding, and for many women, breast tenderness is one of the earliest symptoms of pregnancy. The breasts, which do not fully mature in women until breastfeeding has been initiated, consist of glandular cells arranged in clusters called alveoli, within which there are acini, or milk-producing cells (see Fig. 7.3a, b). The alveoli branch into ducts spreading throughout the breasts and leading to the area behind the nipple where they bulge out to provide a reservoir, or ampulla, for milk. Small contractile cells, termed myoepithelial cells, surround the acini cells, which, under the influence of hormones in the postnatal period, squeeze the milk from the acini cells into the ducts and assist in propelling it towards the ampullae and nipple. The nipple is sensitive erectile tissue with about 15–20 openings from the ampullae to allow milk to be expelled. The pigmented area, called the areola, has sebaceous duct openings to lubricate the surface; these are called Montgomery's tubercles. The breasts are served by a rich blood supply that increases in pregnancy and during lactation but, apart from the nipple, there is a poor nerve supply. The size of the breasts is dictated by the amount of adipose or fat tissue, but does not usually affect the ability of the mother to breastfeed.

The preparation of the breasts begins very early in pregnancy with the development of the blood supply, acini cells and lactiferous ducts, which all combine to cause tenderness and discomfort. This must be taken into account when carrying out back massage with the mother lying prone, which may squash the tissues and cause pain; support under the curve formed by the chin, anterior neck and upper surface of the breast may be helpful.

From about 16 weeks of pregnancy there may be some leakage of clear fluid from the breasts as the colostrum, or early nutritious pre-milk, begins

Fig. 7.3. *(a) Anatomy of the breast (sagittal section).*

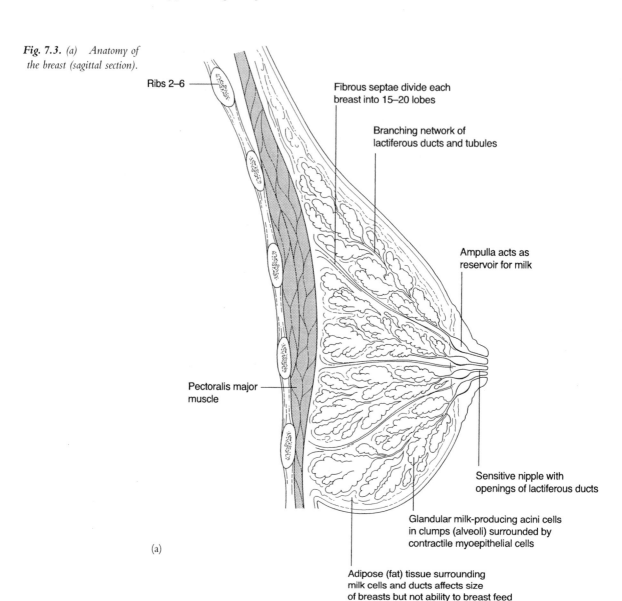

Ribs 2–6

Fibrous septae divide each
breast into 15–20 lobes

Branching network of
lactiferous ducts and tubules

Ampulla acts as
reservoir for milk

Pectoralis major
muscle

Sensitive nipple with
openings of lactiferous ducts

Glandular milk-producing acini cells
in clumps (alveoli) surrounded by
contractile myoepithelial cells

(a)

Adipose (fat) tissue surrounding
milk cells and ducts affects size
of breasts but not ability to breast feed

to develop; in pregnancy its function is to clear the ducts in readiness for
the new milk after delivery. This may be a source of embarrassment to the
mother during aromatherapy treatments, and hygiene for other clients
should be considered if soiling of couch covers occurs.

Breast and nipple self-massage may be suggested antenatally to mothers,
both to prepare them for labour and breastfeeding, and to stimulate lactation after delivery. Breast massage is performed gently, working towards the
nipple; it encourages the mother to become accustomed to handling her
breasts before lactation. Massage from the axilla to the nipple can facilitate
milk flow and prevent stasis.

Fig. 7.3. (b) Frontal view of the breast.

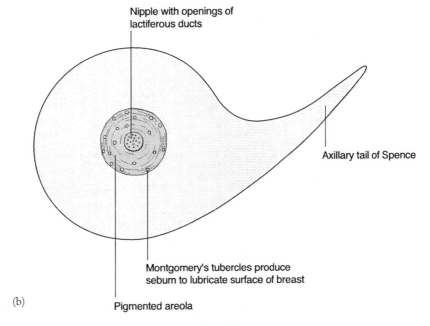

(b)

Fig. 7.3. (c) Physiology of lactation.

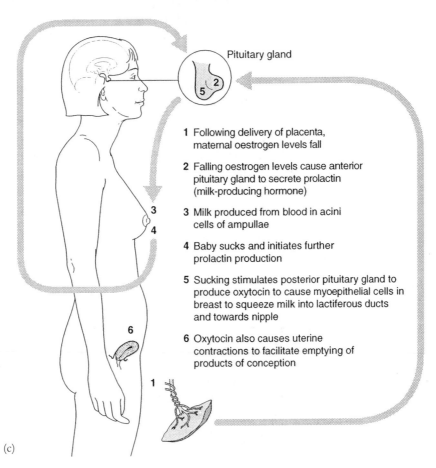

Pituitary gland

1 Following delivery of placenta, maternal oestrogen levels fall

2 Falling oestrogen levels cause anterior pituitary gland to secrete prolactin (milk-producing hormone)

3 Milk produced from blood in acini cells of ampullae

4 Baby sucks and initiates further prolactin production

5 Sucking stimulates posterior pituitary gland to produce oxytocin to cause myoepithelial cells in breast to squeeze milk into lactiferous ducts and towards nipple

6 Oxytocin also causes uterine contractions to facilitate emptying of products of conception

(c)

Nipple massage, rolling the nipple between thumb and forefinger, can be carried out daily in the last 4 weeks of pregnancy to stimulate oxytocin production which will help to ripen the cervix in preparation for labour, harden the nipples for breastfeeding and promote a good supply of milk. Mothers should be advised to massage only one nipple at a time, for about 5 minutes, as bilateral stimulation could precipitate hypertonic uterine action.

Following delivery of the hormone-rich placenta after the birth of the baby, the mother's levels of oestrogen and progesterone fall, which allows a surge in pituitary prolactin, the hormone responsible for the production of milk, from fatty globules in the blood, within the acini cells (see Fig. 7.3c). Sucking of the baby at the breast triggers a neurohormonal reflex that causes oxytocin to be released from the pituitary gland. This results in contracting of the myoepithelial cells, which squeeze the acini cells so that milk is pushed into the lactiferous ducts and towards the nipple. A second hormonal cycle is stimulated by the baby's sucking, which produces more prolactin and more milk. A supply and demand situation is thus in action, and by far the best means of encouraging a good supply of milk is by frequent feeding of the baby on demand; conversely, for those women unable or unwilling to breast-feed, the most appropriate method of suppressing lactation is the physio-logical one in which there is no further stimulation of the breasts.

Aromatherapy oils or herbal teas can, however, help the mother who is breastfeeding. Essential oils classified as galactogues (increasing lactation) can be used to stimulate milk production and include aniseed, basil, caraway, dill, fennel, and lemongrass. Any direct application of essential oils to the breasts in massage or in the bath should be rinsed off before putting the baby to the breast to avoid ingestion, but many of these, notably fennel or dill, can be drunk as a tea throughout the puerperium.

When the milk supply is poor, stimulation of the reflexology breast zones on the feet can be attempted (Fig. 7.4a). Rather than carry out spe-cific reflexology techniques, the midwife can gently massage these areas and advise the mother to rub the corresponding hand zones intermittently (Fig. 7.4b). There is a theory that women who have had an intravenous infusion, sited in the dorsum of the hand during labour, may have impaired lactation, and this would be well worth investigating. The shiatsu points P1 and St16 can also be stimulated to promote lactation (Fig. 7.4c).

For engorgement of the breasts, the application of cabbage leaves pro-duces, in many women, spectacular results. Dark green cabbage leaves are wiped clean and cooled in the refrigerator then applied to engorged breasts. Often within seconds the leaves become wet, when they should be removed and replaced with new leaves, this process being repeated until relief is obtained. Women who have employed this method of relieving engorgement are amazed at the results despite their initial scepticism, and it provides an inexpensive means of treatment without any known side-effects.

Fig. 7.4. *(a) Foot reflex zone therapy to stimulate lactation. (b) Hand reflex zones to massage to encourage lactation. (From Tiran & Mack 2000 with permission.) (c) Shiatsu points to stimulate lactation.*

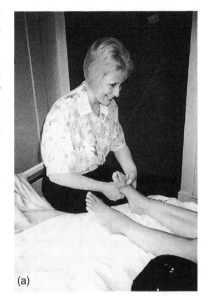

(a)

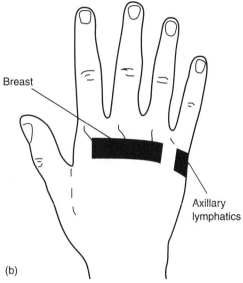

Breast

Axillary lymphatics

(b)

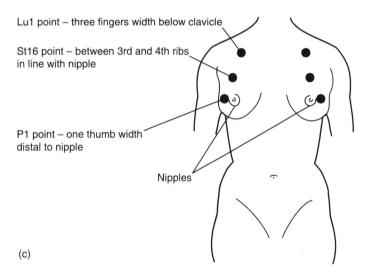

Lu1 point – three fingers width below clavicle

St16 point – between 3rd and 4th ribs in line with nipple

P1 point – one thumb width distal to nipple

Nipples

(c)

Suppression of lactation has been achieved with jasmine flowers. Shrivastav et al (1988) demonstrated a reduction in serum prolactin levels in women who had had jasmine flowers applied to the breasts, and the earlier work of Abraham et al (1979) suggested that pituitary inhibition occurs as a result of an olfactory pathway to the hypothalamus. This does bring into question the use of jasmine to stimulate lactation, as suggested in some aromatherapy texts, although it may be that the essential oil acts as a *regulator*, not specifically as a stimulant or suppressant.

Similarly, Tisserand (1992, p. 298) suggested that geranium may be useful as a means of reducing the flow of milk, yet Worwood (1990, p. 282) has advocated geranium to stimulate lactation. Alternative suppressants include peppermint, for example using a cold compress soaked in water and oil of peppermint, although this must be washed off before feeding the baby.

Sore nipples may respond to the direct application of geranium leaves or the use of a cream to which has been added a few drops of geranium essential oil. Calendula essential oil is recommended by some authorities but there are several proprietary brands of calendula creams which can be used rather than making one's own. Camomile has also been used both in essential oil form and as a proprietary cream (Kamillosan). A simple home remedy for sore nipples is to steep camomile teabags in boiled water, drain, cool and then apply them to the nipples, keeping them in place with the bra.

If the mother shows signs and symptoms of mastitis or a developing breast abscess, a compress of tea tree oil is the most effective method of combating infection; alternatively geranium essential oil can be used.

Bruising

By far the best treatment for severe bruising, particularly of the perineum and/or buttocks following delivery, is arnica, a homoeopathic preparation and one of the few that is universally appropriate for trauma. It is available in both cream and tablet form, although the cream should not be applied to an open wound such as a perineal suture line. Tablets should be taken immediately after the birth and at 4-hourly intervals thereafter until the symptoms subside, usually about 3 days. Arnica is included here because it should be the first line of treatment and a normal part of maternity care. Midwives should take action to introduce it into their units by stimulating discussion with medical and managerial colleagues and presenting sufficient evidence to convince them of the benefits of a trial period. Homoeopathic arnica can be given safely in pregnancy, for example when a large contusion has developed after a difficult venepuncture, but the essential oil is contraindicated completely in aromatherapy.

There are some essential oils that can be valuable for bruising, the safest of which is lavender, from the third trimester onwards. If this is used in a bath or bidet it may also help perineal healing following delivery, while oil of black pepper added to the bidet or massaged into the skin can relieve the discomfort of bruised buttocks. Other oils effective in dealing with bruising are not considered safe during pregnancy and include fennel, hyssop, mint and parsley.

Caesarean section

Although it may not be appropriate to use essential oils during the operative procedure, there are several ways in which aromatherapy can be of help to women around this time, particularly if the Caesarean is planned. Massage with essential oils in the weeks leading up to the operation may assist in relaxing the mother; occasionally, where the indication for the Caesarean is a breech presentation of the fetus, *gentle* clockwise abdominal massage may relax the mother sufficiently to encourage spontaneous fetal cephalic version, although the mother should not rely on this – there are other complementary therapies that may be more effective (see Tiran & Mack 2000).

In cases of hypertension necessitating operative delivery, massage and essential oils could be used to reduce the blood pressure, even if only temporarily, and as a treatment shortly before surgery can be an appropriate natural premedication, although consideration should be given to possible interactions with drugs.

Essential oils such as lavender and tea tree may be offered in baths as a preventative measure against postoperative uterine, respiratory, urinary tract or abdominal wound infection. Hammer, Carson & Riley's research (1996) suggests that tea tree may be effective in removing transient skin flora while suppressing but retaining resident flora. Much other research into tea tree oil (see entry for Tea tree in Chapter 8) abundantly supports its use as both a preventative and curative oil against infections.

In relation to the prevention of other postoperative complications, there are two research projects that appear to suggest that clove oil may act as an antithrombotic agent (Saeed & Gilani 1994) and that a combination of high doses of vitamin A and citral, a constituent of many essential oils, may reduce the formation of peritoneal adhesions (Demetriou et al 1974).

Postoperative pain relief may be achieved with essential oils once the acute phase requiring intravenous, spinal or intramuscular analgesics has passed, or possibly in conjunction with some medications. Lavender, with its various terpenes, is both analgesic and sedative; when inhaled it will also aid respiratory function and possibly prevent upper respiratory tract infection. Atanassova-Shopova & Roussinov (1970) tested *Lavandula vera* D.C. (a type of lavender oil) and found that it potentiated narcotic effects, perhaps indicating a possible interaction with morphine, pethidine and other narcotics. Dale & Cornwell's trial (1994) investigating the use of lavender for postnatal perineal care failed to demonstrate wound-healing capabilities of the oil, but did show a statistically significant result in reducing discomfort.

The mother may welcome aromatherapy massages of her back, legs, neck and shoulders or full body once she is up and coping with the effects both of delivering her baby and of having a major abdominal operation; the long-term sequelae of the latter should not be underestimated.

Carpal tunnel syndrome	See Oedema, p. 102.

Conjunctivitis	Newborn babies occasionally develop conjunctivitis, although infective conjunctivitis is less common than a simple moist eye, usually caused by blocked tear ducts. As the eye is a sensitive area of the body, it is necessary to ensure that medical advice is sought as soon as possible to eliminate

more serious problems, but where the baby (or mother) suffers from true conjunctivitis aromatherapy principles can be of use. It is important to remember, however, that essential oils should *never* be used on the eyes even when they are well diluted. The simplest and safest management is to irrigate the eye with a solution of camomile tea, with its soothing, anti-inflammatory and antiseptic properties. Rose is thought to be effective and can be applied in the form of an eye compress soaked in rosewater, but camomile is usually more easily available.

Constipation and colic

A variety of factors contribute to the high incidence of constipation in pregnant and newly delivered mothers, and in their infants. The action of progesterone in relaxing the gastrointestinal tract and slowing peristalsis provides a physiological reason for gestational difficulties with defaecation, often compounded by the unnecessary use of regular iron administration, although this practice, fortunately, is on the decline. A high intake of tea (tannin) will also exacerbate the condition. The traditional practice of restricting food intake during labour (although less so now), together with poor postnatal nutrition for many mothers in hospital, adds to the problem, as does the reflex inhibition from which many mothers suffer if there is perineal trauma. Appropriate nutritional advice is the best means of prevention: plenty of fresh fruit and vegetables to provide fibre, and a fluid intake of at least 3 litres a day.

The easiest and most effective treatment is firm clockwise abdominal massage, carried out for about 5 minutes, and/or clockwise massage of the arches of the feet. The latter works on the reflex zones to the gastro-intestinal tract and may be easier on heavily pregnant women. It is not feasible to perform abdominal massage on a mother who has had a Caesarean section, but *gentle* clockwise massage of the foot arches may produce results (Fig. 7.5).

The mother can be directed to perform intermittent self-shiatsu on the CV6 point. She should lie on her back and press deeply to a depth of about one inch, then maintain the pressure for a few minutes while breathing deeply. The LI11 point can also be worked, and postnatally the LI4 point, although this is contraindicated during pregnancy (Fig. 7.6).

If the neonate becomes constipated the same gentle clockwise abdominal and foot arch massage can be carried out, by the mother. Similarly when the baby suffers from colic, abdominal massage will stimulate peristalsis so that the air bubbles will be pushed along the intestines and expelled via the rectum. It is best to show the mother how to do it herself, for a fretful baby often leads to a distressed mother, and the action of performing the massage may help in calming her. Camomile tea can be given on a teaspoon, flavoured with honey if necessary.

Some aromatherapy research has been conducted into the antispasmodic actions of some essential oils. Perfumi et al (1995) showed a dose-dependent spasmolytic activity of essential oil of *Artemesia thuscula* on

Fig. 7.5. *Reflex zones for the gastrointestinal tract. Note the direction of the intestines: clockwise massage of the foot arches will treat constipation.*

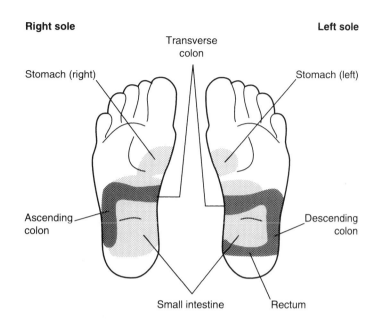

Right sole   **Left sole**

Transverse colon

Stomach (right)   Stomach (left)

Ascending colon   Descending colon

Small intestine   Rectum

Fig. 7.6. *Shiatsu points for constipation.*

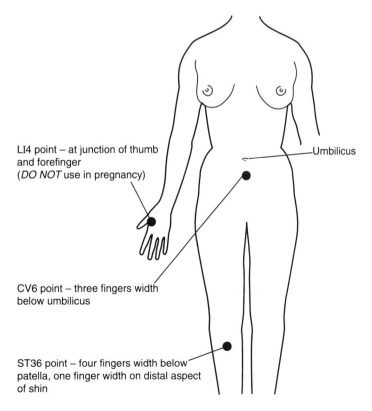

LI4 point – at junction of thumb and forefinger (*DO NOT* use in pregnancy)

Umbilicus

CV6 point – three fingers width below umbilicus

ST36 point – four fingers width below patella, one finger width on distal aspect of shin

guinea pig ileum and attributed this to the davanone in one chemotype and β-thujone (both ketones) in the other chemotype. Ketones were also found to be partially responsible for the antispasmodic activity of *Artemesia herba* in earlier research by Yashphe et al (1987). Antispasmodic action of *Achillea ageratum* on rat duodenum (de la Puerta & Herrera 1995) was demonstrated by the inhibition of acetylcholine and barium chloride-induced contractions. Contractions induced by acetylcholine, as well as histamine, potassium and calcium ions, were also inhibited by the essential oil of *Croton zehntneri*, mainly by the constituents of estragole and to a lesser extent anethole (phenols), although it was noted that the whole essential oil was more effective than either of the constituents in isolation (Coelho-de-Souza et al 1997). The relatively newly recognized New Zealand essential oils of manuka and kanuka were found to be spasmolytic and spasmogenic respectively (Lis-Balchin et al 1996a). Various chemotypes of *Thymus* have also shown spasmolytic activity: *Thymus membranaceus* (Zarzuelo et al 1987); *Thymus granatensis* and *T. zygis* (thyme oil) (Cabo et al 1986); *T. vulgaris* (thyme) (Rangelov 1989); and *T. baeticus* Boiss (Cruz et al 1989).

Among the more commonly used essential oils, *Matricaria chamomilla* may be spasmolytic (Achterrath-Tuckerman et al 1980), although Lis-Balchin et al (1996b) were not able to substantiate this claim. Cardamom oil (Al-Zuhair et al 1996) and various types of pelargonium (Lis-Balchin et al 1995) have been shown to be spasmolytic. Ginger appears to have a cholagogic effect on the colon (Ozaki & Soedigdo 1988). Rosemary has also been found to be mildly spasmolytic (Giachetti et al 1988, Taddei et al 1988) although Hof & Ammon (1989) postulate that both the complete essential oil and its major constituent, 1,8-cineole, have a greater spasmolytic effect on cardiac muscle than on intestinal muscle.

However, peppermint and other members of the mint family appear to be the clear winners in their effects on the gastrointestinal tract, either by direct antispasmodic activity or by influencing bile secretion (Duthie 1981, Giachetti et al 1988, Hardcastle et al 1996, Hills & Aaronson 1991, Leicester & Hunt 1982, Rangelov 1989, Rangelov et al 1988, Rees et al 1979, Somerville et al 1984, Trabace et al 1992). Citrus oils have long been quoted in aromatherapy texts as being effective in treating constipation, although there appears to be very little research into these oils; suffice it to say that, in the knowledge that they are safe to use in pregnancy, they may be suitable oils to administer, either alone or in combination, for abdominal massage.

Expectant and newly delivered mothers may like to drink camomile tea and to increase the amount of citrus fruit in the diet. Postnatally a massage with a blend of orange, grapefruit, nutmeg and camomile, applied to the abdomen in a clockwise direction and to the sacral area of the lower back, can work wonders.

Depression Hormonal upheavals, especially in the postnatal period, can lead to depression of varying severity. Many women experience the 'blues' about 3–4 days after delivery and quickly recover. Others develop the condition within the first 6 weeks after the birth; some will have a low-grade depression that they are able to deal with themselves, and some will require short- or long-term psychiatric support. A few women develop depression during pregnancy, although many more feel a variety of emotions such as anxiety, fear and stress.

The emotional symptoms of depression may take many forms, including fear and anxiety, panic, paranoia, impatience, apathy and irritability, and various essential oils can be utilized to combat these symptoms.

Various essential oils have been found to have sedative effects that may be helpful in promoting sleep and rest, with the pharmacological action being attributed to linalool, especially in neroli (Elisabetsky et al 1995, Jager et al 1992). Lavender may be useful in low doses towards term and postnatally to encourage sleep (Dunn et al 1995) and to aid relaxation (Buchbauer et al 1993, Imberger et al 1993, Karamat et al 1992, Ludvigson & Rottman 1989, Sugano & Sato 1991), although Buchbauer et al (1991) considered that lavandula chemotypes with a high level of 1,8-cineole may be more excitory than sedative. Sweet fennel (*Foeniculum vulgarae*) has been shown to reduce stress and fatigue, probably due to reduced excitation of parasympathetic nerves (Nagai et al 1991), but should only be used following delivery. Conversely sweet orange oil was found to increase parasympathetic activity but to effect a positive mood change (Miyazaki et al 1991), as did bitter orange oil (Miyake et al 1991). Sweet orange, and other citral and citronellal-containing essential oils may be refreshing, although Takeuchi et al (1991) noticed a gender-related difference in the mood effects of these constituents and other oils, and Warm & Dember (1990) found similar gender differences on vigilance performance and stress when administering peppermint and muguet. Ylang ylang, sandalwood, bergamot and other citrus oils such as grapefruit, lime, mandarin and tangerine may be pleasant and safe additions to a blend for relaxation.

Although it is not the purpose of this book to cover other types of complementary and natural remedies, Bach flower remedies may be extremely useful and effective (see Tiran & Mack 2000). There is, of course, no replacement for listening and counselling, but in severe cases this should only be attempted by midwives, health visitors, doctors or therapists with the appropriate qualifications.

A full body massage, if there is time and the mother wishes it, may be a wonderfully pampering means of allowing her some time for herself and facilitate a reduction in the negative feelings she is experiencing; alternatively a back or neck and shoulder massage can be helpful. Vaporization of the essential oils into the room is another way of refreshing the mother, or she could relax by adding the appropriate oils to the bath.

Jane was a professional woman who had recently left a demanding career. She had initially been upset when she discovered she was pregnant but gradually accepted the fact, and was pleased on account of her husband who was Italian and 'over the moon' about the impending birth. However, as term approached Jane became increasingly anxious and noticeably depressed about her imagined inability to give birth and to care for the baby, and this was made worse by her husband's lack of understanding and insistence that her negative attitude was spoiling a wonderful experience for him. Eventually Jane was admitted to the antenatal ward for psychiatric referral.

The midwife-aromatherapist was able to see Jane for several consecutive days and offered a foot massage for stress relief, which she gratefully accepted. A combination of ylang ylang, mandarin and frankincense was used and Jane reported feeling much better after each massage, and was able to sleep. While this treatment was only palliative and in no way treated the cause, it did help Jane to feel calmer and gave her the opportunity to talk about her concerns.

Diarrhoea   Causative factors in cases of diarrhoea are complex, ranging from diet to stress, infective organisms and, in pregnancy, hormonal effects. Midwives will in the course of their work be able to give relevant dietary advice to mothers. Diarrhoea of infective aetiology requires medical care, although there are many essential oils that have proven antibacterial, antiviral and antifungal properties, notably tea tree. In addition to any prescribed medication, the mother could be encouraged to soak in a bath containing tea tree oil, with sufficient water to cover the abdomen, or a compress could be applied to the lower abdomen and sacrum.

When the diarrhoea is stress related, anti-anxiety essential oils should be used in synergy with antispasmodic oils. Neroli and petitgrain can be effective, while sandalwood has long been recognized in Ayurvedic medicine as a treatment for diarrhoea. Although both neroli and sandalwood are expensive, the synergistic effects of blending them together make them extremely beneficial for mothers with this problem. Camomile essential oil has also been found to have antispasmodic actions (Achterrath-Tuckermann et al 1980). Later research (Taddei et al 1988) compared the spasmolytic (antispasmodic) actions of peppermint, sage and rosemary oils in animals and found the effects to be similar with all three oils. Rosemary's actions were attributed to the level of pinene and borneol, and it was thought that it worked by antagonizing acetylcholine Rosemary, therefore, may be used with caution in late pregnancy, except in women with raised blood pressure, but sage is contraindicated (see also p. 86, Constipation, for further research into the spasmolytic and spasmogenic effects of essential oils).

Fig. 7.7.   Shiatsu points to relieve diarrhoea.

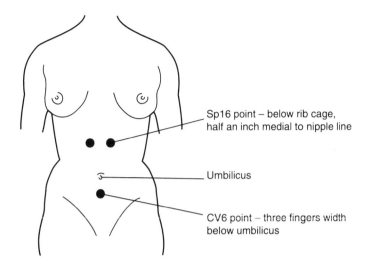

Sp16 point – below rib cage, half an inch medial to nipple line

Umbilicus

CV6 point – three fingers width below umbilicus

The essential oils can be administered as an abdominal massage, which should be *anti*clockwise to slow down peristalsis, or a compress can be applied to the suprapubic area. Similarly, anticlockwise massage of the arches of the feet will work on the reflex zones for the gastrointestinal tract (Fig. 7.7), and the practitioner can incorporate shiatsu pressure to the LV2 point. The mother can also be advised to press on the two Sp16 points on the abdomen.

If diarrhoea occurs immediately before or during labour, which is not uncommon, essential oils can be used to freshen and cleanse the mother, perhaps added to the bidet for a vulval wash; this will have the added benefit of preventing contamination by faeces of the vulval and perineal areas. Any of the above oils may be used according to the mother's preference.

Care should be taken if a baby develops diarrhoea as this may be due to gastroenteritis or an undiagnosed condition of the digestive tract. However, if it appears that the baby has simply responded adversely to something the mother may have eaten to excess (e.g. chocolate), anticlockwise abdominal massage with a 1% blend of camomile or mandarin may help to slow down peristalsis. It should be stressed here that breast-fed babies rarely suffer diarrhoea as a result of maternal diet and that mothers should continue to eat a well-balanced diet containing normal amounts of fruit and vegetables. Consequently practitioners should seek medical advice in cases of true neonatal diarrhoea (as opposed to loose stools).

Epilepsy   It is unlikely that midwives or aromatherapists will use essential oils to treat pregnant women with epilepsy as they will be under strict medical supervision in order to monitor the ways in which pregnancy may alter the incidence or severity of fits, and their effects on fetal and maternal wellbeing. It would indeed be irresponsible to do so without the knowledge and approval of the consultant obstetrician and physician. However, there may be some individuals in whom a fit is triggered by stress, fear, panic or anger, and it might be appropriate to offer regular massage with a safe anticonvulsive essential oil such as lavender (from the third trimester) or one that is suitable for relieving stress and anxiety, e.g. orange or ylang ylang, on condition that the aromas themselves do not precipitate fits.

Research in an epilepsy clinic with ten (non-pregnant) patients has shown that, after an initial period of regular massage with a single relaxing essential oil, patients can be taught to associate the aroma alone with a sense of relaxation and, in conjunction with autohypnosis, can use this as a countermeasure to prevent a fit occurring (Betts 1994). It is interesting to note that most of these ten patients chose ylang ylang as their preferred olfactory countermeasure; in a few subjects, in whom an increase in arousal suppressed the onset of a fit, an alerting oil such as lemongrass was chosen.

There are sufficient data from aromatherapy research to demonstrate without doubt that essential oils and their aromas can have a variety of effects on the central nervous sytem. This must be considered when caring for women who are known epileptics, but must also be borne in mind if the oils are used on those with a predisposition to fits, either through a genetic tendency or in cases of pre-eclampsia. Contingent negative variation, or slow brain wave responses, have been shown either to increase or decrease following exposure to a range of oils (Manley 1993). Lavender was thought to have a neurodepressive effect (Guillemain et al 1989) and to be a sedative (Buchbauer et al 1993, Imberger et al 1993, Karamat et al 1992, Sugano 1989), although Lorig & Roberts (1990) found it to be highly arousing and distracting. Early research by Atanassova-Shopova & Roussinov (1970) showed that lavender oil was anticonvulsive and potentiated the effects of narcotics; this was replicated by Yamada et al (1994). Lemongrass is also neurodepressive, acting similarly to tranquillizers (Seth et al 1976), while jasmine has been shown to be excitory (Karamat et al 1992, Kikuchi et al 1989, Sugano 1989, Sugano & Sato 1991). α- and β-santalol, constituents of sandalwood oil, are thought to produce sedative effects but not to be anticonvulsant (Okugawa et al 1995), whereas bergamot oil is both sedative and anticonvulsant (Occhiuto et al 1995).

It is important in maternity care to differentiate between epileptic and eclamptic fits, although the management of fits of any aetiology is the same and, during pregnancy, revolves around preserving maternal and fetal life.

When using essential oils generally for childbearing women it is necessary to be aware of oils that may initiate epileptic fits; these include rosemary, fennel, hyssop, sage and wormwood. In rosemary, this may be due to the ketone, camphor (Steinmetz et al 1987), which has long been reported as causing epileptiform fits if taken in sufficient quantity (Craig 1953, Rubin et al 1949). Of these, only rosemary and fennel are likely to be used for this client group but they should be avoided in anyone with a personal or family history of epilepsy, hypertension or pre-eclampsia. Davis (1988, p. 119) suggests that minute amounts of rosemary may be helpful for epileptics, in a homoeopathic manner. This is supported by Asjes (1993), an aromatherapist experienced in the use of essential oils for epileptic children who has administered rosemary to very apathetic clients.

Epistaxis Nosebleeds are not uncommon in pregnancy due to hypervolaemia, and capillary and vasodilatation. Essential oil of lemon acts as a haemostatic agent and can be used as a glabellary compress; alternatively a small gauze swab soaked in water to which has been added fresh lemon juice or the essential oil can be gently inserted into the nostril. If the epistaxis is associated with hypertension, lavender may also be used from the end of pregnancy.

Hair care Pregnant and newly delivered women often experience changes in the condition or growth of their hair: some find that it becomes more greasy, others that it feels very dry; many women lose hair, especially in the months after the birth of the baby. Aromatherapy has much to offer mothers at this time, although they should be advised not to use the same essential oils consistently. The normal safeguards concerning essential oil use during pregnancy should be adhered to, for absorption through the scalp occurs as with other areas of the body.

For greasy hair the mother could use essential oil of lemon or petit-grain in early pregnancy, but, if she is not hypertensive, the most effective oil from the third trimester onwards is rosemary. Two or three drops of essential oil can be added to the rinsing water, or fresh lemon juice squeezed into the bowl; sprigs of fresh rosemary are safe to use and can be just as beneficial to the hair. A few drops of patchouli may also be used.

Camomile can be useful for hair that has been previously permed or coloured or which has become very fragile. Incidentally, most hairdressers would advise women to refrain from having a perm at this time as they are often unsuccessful, possibly due to hormonal influences.

Dry hair may respond to rosemary, geranium or sandalwood, with lavender being a useful alternative after 28 weeks' gestation. Blending the essential oils into a rich nourishing base oil such as jojoba or avocado can enhance their action.

Hair loss more commonly seems to occur in the postnatal period and can be treated with oils such as rosemary, rose, camomile, lemon, cypress, clary sage or calendula. Lime, lemon, mandarin and rosemary may help dandruff, as may thyme, although antepartum use of the latter is contraindicated.

Regular head massage, without oil, can stimulate and invigorate the scalp and may improve the condition of the hair.

Haemorrhoids Varicose veins in the rectum and anus can be extremely painful, especially if they prolapse as they may do towards the end of pregnancy or after defaecation. Essential oils which act as an astringent and vasoconstrictor may help to relieve pain, including cypress, juniper and frankincense. These may be applied diluted as a compress, or added to a shallow bath or bidet as a local soak. Irritation and itching may be eased by using patchouli or geranium in a similar way. The mother can also be encouraged to eat plenty of garlic to aid the circulatory system in general. Ryman (1991, p. 282) recommends boiling leeks and freezing ice cubes from the cooking water, which can be rubbed on to the afflicted area for immediate relief.

Headaches

Headaches are suffered by many women in the first trimester as a result of cerebral vasodilatation, and again towards term in some, in association with hypertension. Head massage (without oils) to stimulate the scalp and cerebral circulation may ease discomfort. A 'hairwashing' action is used to massage the scalp firmly. Massage has been compared favourably with other treatments for headaches of variable aetiology (Jenson et al 1990).

Peppermint has been shown to be effective in treating headaches, and in conjunction with eucalyptus, has a relaxing but not an analgesic effect; eucalyptus alone does not relieve pain (Gobel et al 1994, 1995). Occhiuto et al (1995) found bergamot to be an effective analgesic, and lemongrass and its major constituent, myrcene, appear to be pain-relieving (Lorenzetti et al 1991, Paumgartten et al 1990), although the effects of myrcene on the liver and stomach in mice indicate that it should not be administered orally. Peri- and postnatal developmental toxicity in rats exposed to β-myrcene indicate caution, although Delgado et al (1993a) suggest that toxic dose levels were unlikely to be attained in humans. Work by Moran et al (1989) showed analgesic effects of a variety of *Artemesia* essential oil, while cardamom oil compares favourably with aspirin, although it may be contraindicated in pregnancy owing to a high level of 1,8-cineole (ketone, up to 60%; Al-Zuhair et al 1996). Aboutabl & Abdelhakim (1996) suggest that certain types of *Melaleuca* grown in Egypt may also possess analgesic properties, while a Brazilian herb, rotundifolone, may also reduce pain (Almeida et al 1996). The analgesic effects of several Turkish oils tested by Aydin et al (1996) are thought to be due to the carvacrol content.

Incorporating shiatsu can enhance the effects of simple massage, working specifically on shiatsu points GV16, GV24.5 and St3. In a trial by Puustjarvi et al (1990) acupressure was used successfully in conjunction with head massage for 21 subjects with chronic tension headaches.

Other shiatsu points found on the feet can be incorporated into reflexology and include LV3 and GB41 (Fig. 7.9). Reflexology first aid may also be effective in sedating the pain. The carer should ascertain exactly where in the head the mother is experiencing pain and then relate this to the appropriate zone on the big toes. By gentle pressure around these zones a painful spot will be elicited; the carer should press firmly on the epicentre of this painful spot until the pain in the toe has gone. If the headache

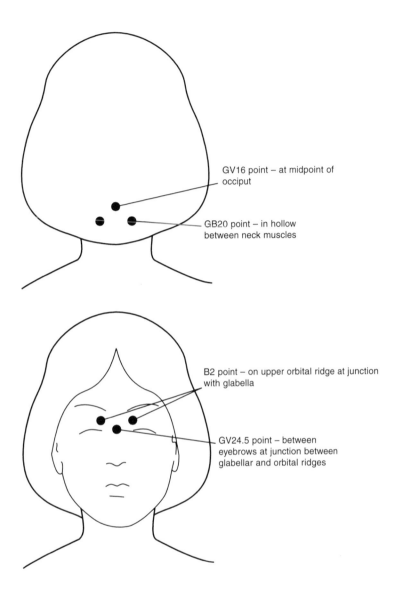

Fig. 7.8.   *Shiatsu points to relieve headaches.*

GV16 point – at midpoint of occiput

GB20 point – in hollow between neck muscles

B2 point – on upper orbital ridge at junction with glabella

GV24.5 point – between eyebrows at junction between glabellar and orbital ridges

is unilateral, only the big toe on the same side as the headache is treated; if it is bilateral then both big toes are treated (Fig. 7.9).

Shiatsu massage of the head including the GV19, GV20, GV21, GV24.5, GB20 and B10 points can be very relaxing and relieve associated headaches, and a general reflexology treatment may also help (Fig. 7.8).

Miranda had suffered headaches with no identified aetiology from early in her pregnancy, and found they were relieved by resting. As she was receiving regular reflex zone therapy for stress throughout pregnancy she mentioned to her therapist that they were more frequent at about 30 weeks' gestation, although her blood pressure was normal and she had no oedema or proteinuria. The reflex zone therapist, one of the midwives in the materity unit, was able to treat Miranda for her headaches by working on her feet, with some success.

Following a normal delivery at term, Miranda again began to suffer the headaches, and this time the therapist used a combination of zone therapy and head massage. On one occasion the therapist saw Miranda while she was actually experiencing a severe headache, and applied lavender and peppermint oils to her temples, which brought a rapid response. No cause was found for the symptom and gradually the headaches subsided, probably indicating a reaction to fluctuating hormone levels, but the treatment did at least make Miranda feel more relaxed, which in itself may have helped.

Fig. 7.9. *Shiatsu points and reflex zones on the feet to treat headache.*

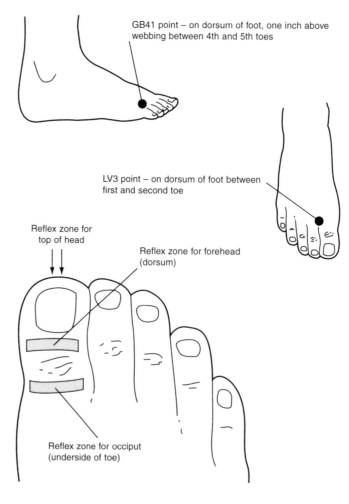

GB41 point – on dorsum of foot, one inch above webbing between 4th and 5th toes

LV3 point – on dorsum of foot between first and second toe

Reflex zone for top of head

Reflex zone for forehead (dorsum)

Reflex zone for occiput (underside of toe)

Heartburn and indigestion

In the second and third trimesters of pregnancy, heartburn may become a problem for some women owing to the increased weight and consequent pressure effects, coupled with the relaxing action of progesterone on the cardiac sphincter of the stomach.

Increased acidity in the stomach may respond to the use of lemon, either by recommending that the woman makes a lemon cordial or by gentle back and abdominal massage using the essential oil. One might assume that the acidic nature of lemon means it is contraindicated, but it appears to work by neutralization of the citric acid, especially during digestion, resulting in the production of alkaline carbonates of calcium and potassium.

Judicious use of essential oil of black pepper in a blend with orange or mandarin can help, as may frankincense. Near term, when the use of lavender and marjoram in small amounts is not thought to be a problem, abdominal massage with a blend of these, or of lavender and camomile, can also be effective.

The carminative properties of fennel and peppermint make these two of the best plants to use for indigestion and heartburn in normal circumstances, but in pregnancy fennel should be avoided. Teas of camomile or ginger may be best. Increasing the amount of garlic in the diet assists in reducing acidity and aiding digestion; this may depend on whether the mother likes the taste, especially at a time when the senses of taste and smell may be altered.

The use of choleretic essential oils, i.e. those that stimulate bile production, should be considered towards term or in the postnatal period. Nerol has been shown, in rats and guinea pigs, to have choleretic effects (Rangelov et al 1988) and is found in essential oils of neroli, petitgrain and orange.

Induction or acceleration of labour

It must be stressed here that induction of labour should *not* be attempted by anyone other than a member of the conventional obstetric team. It is not appropriate for non-medically qualified therapists to attempt to interfere in an essentially normal physiological process. However, although not normally the province of the midwife, it may be acceptable on occasions, in consultation with the obstetricians, for manual techniques to be used in an attempt to initiate or accelerate labour. Conversely it is important to know which techniques should not be used during pregnancy in case they inadvertently cause labour to commence. For aromatherapists who are not midwives, oils that aid relaxation can be used if the mother has simply gone past her due date.

Various shiatsu points can be stimulated to induce uterine action and to relieve contraction pain, including the GB21, LI4, B167, K3 and GB27–GB34 points. (Fig. 7.10), although research in 1987 by Lyrenas et al suggests that prenatal *acupuncture*, rather than acupressure, may prolong the duration of both pregnancy and labour. Regular stimulation of the

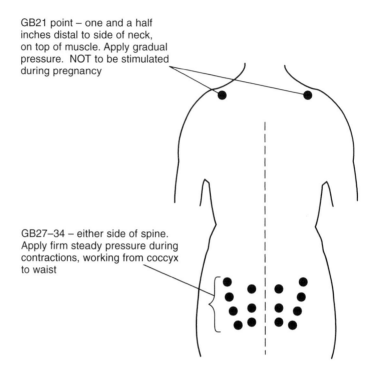

Fig. 7.10. Shiatsu points for labour.

GB21 point – one and a half inches distal to side of neck, on top of muscle. Apply gradual pressure. NOT to be stimulated during pregnancy

GB27–34 – either side of spine. Apply firm steady pressure during contractions, working from coccyx to waist

B167 point using the acupuncture technique of moxibustion has also been shown to be effective in changing a breech to a cephalic presentation (Beal 1992, Budd 1992).

Reflexology to the foot zones for the uterus and the pituitary gland can be stimulated to enhance uterine action before, during or after delivery; it can be a particularly effective treatment for retained placenta, especially in situations such as a home birth where there may not be access to additional drugs (Fig. 7.11).

Any of the essential oils that enhance uterine action could theoretically be administered in an attempt to initiate contractions, although it is likely that these will be used to accelerate labour once established. Lavender and jasmine are effective for this purpose. Raspberry leaf tea is advocated by herbalists to tone the uterus before, during and after labour. It may be drunk daily from mid-pregnancy, gradually increasing the amount, and should assist in ripening the cervix, coordinating uterine action in labour and aiding involution in the puerperium.

Insomnia and tiredness

For many women, tiredness is one of the overwhelming symptoms of pregnancy, particularly in the first and second trimesters if they are still working. The body is working hard to provide energy for fetal development and growth, and the woman needs time to adjust to the fluctuating hormone levels. Increased weight, a variety of physical discomforts and an element of anxiety towards the end of pregnancy can all lead to an exacer-

Fig. 7.11. *Reflexology for labour.*

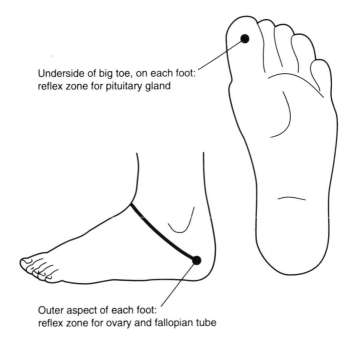

Underside of big toe, on each foot:
reflex zone for pituitary gland

Outer aspect of each foot:
reflex zone for ovary and fallopian tube

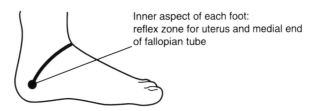

Inner aspect of each foot:
reflex zone for uterus and medial end
of fallopian tube

bation of tiredness and an inability either to go to sleep or to sleep for long periods. Postnatally the mother has to recover physically and psychologically from the birth and learn to cope with the demands of a new baby while her body again undergoes the changes brought about by the endocrine system.

Two of the most commonly used essential oils for helping people to sleep are camomile and lavender: camomile tea may be drunk before retiring. Lavender has been shown to be effective in both inducing and prolonging sleep (Hardy 1991, Henry et al 1994, Hudson 1996). Both of these oils can be offered to women in the postnatal period, although any relaxing oil such as neroli, orange or rose oil can help, as a massage, added to the bathwater or inhaled from a handkerchief or the pillow. Where time permits, and if the mother wishes a massage, with or without essential oils, will go a long way towards making her feel more relaxed, as will reflexology treatment.

Nausea and vomiting

One of the earliest symptoms to alert a woman to possible pregnancy is often nausea, with or without vomiting. This is thought to be due to the hormones oestrogen and chorionic gonadotrophin affecting the blood sugar levels, but is sometimes exacerbated by tiredness, stress and an accompanying loss of appetite. Unfortunately, as sickness is usually a first trimester disorder, many of the essential oils that could be of use are contraindicated during the vital weeks of early fetal cell and organ formation; some mothers may also dislike being touched at this time, so will not wish to receive massage.

A great deal of research has been carried out on the use of acupressure to the Pericardium 6 (P6) point for nausea and vomiting during pregnancy, as well as postoperatively and for patients receiving chemotherapy (Barsoum et al 1990, Belluomini et al 1994, De Aloysio & Penacchioni 1992, Dundee & Yang 1990, Dundee et al 1988, Evans et al 1993, Hyde 1989, Price et al 1991, Stannard 1989). It would appear that acupressure wrist bands (popularly used for motion sickness) can be effective in a significant number of women, and this would be an inexpensive means of treating some clients. The bands cost approximately £7 a pair and are reusable, so it would not be a major expense for a maternity unit to keep a supply for loan. Alternatively, Acumagnets™ are now available for application to the P6 point.

However, some women do not respond to these and for those with true hyperemesis gravidarum it may be too late to use them. A question has also been raised by some midwives about their effects on intravenous lines sited in the dorsum of the hand, although personal experience of the author has not revealed any complications. However, it is certainly worth trying the bands or magnets if the mother will wear them. To position the bands correctly, the length of the mother's inner forearm, from wrist crease to elbow, is divided into 12: this gives 12 Chinese anatomical inches. Measuring two anatomical inches up from the wrist crease, on the inner aspect between the two bones, will locate the mother's P6 point, against which the 'button' inside the wrist band or the Acumagnet™ should be pressed. Alternatively, the mother's fingers can be used to measure two and a half fingers width from the wrist crease, to determine the correct spot (Fig. 7.12).

Reflexology could also be useful in treating gestational sickness. General relaxation techniques should be used together with work on the foot zones for the pituitary gland, hepatorenal and digestive systems. The best essential oils are mandarin, tangerine, sweet orange, lime and grapefruit (as long as the mother is not allergic to citrus fruit), all of which will assist in relaxing her, plus ginger to act as an antiemetic. Peppermint and/or spearmint oils can also be effective and refreshing. However, care should be taken to identify the mother's sensitivity to different aromas. Gentle massage of the back and shoulders, or, if the mother can cope with it, of the abdomen may help to ease both nausea and tension.

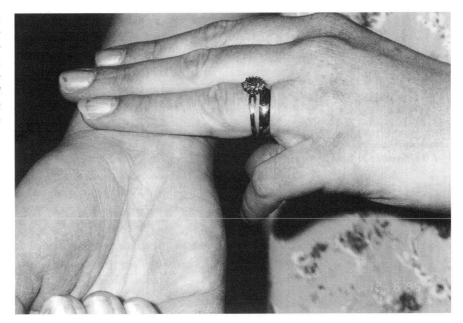

Fig. 7.12. *Identification of P6 acupressure point by the mother. She must use her own finger-breadth (rather than that of the therapist): a slight dip and some tenderness will be felt when the exact point is located.*

Grapefruit is thought to regulate appetite and act as a tonic for the biliary and hepatic systems, particularly in the digestion of fats, so it may be helpful in conjunction with dietary advice for women who are nauseated after eating food with a high fat content. Grapefruit is an especially refreshing essential oil; alternatively, the mother could be encouraged to eat grapefruit regularly during the day – grapefruit contains vitamin B_6 in which some women who suffer sickness may be deficient.

Ginger tea made from a piece of ginger root steeped in boiling water, with honey added to combat hypoglycaemia, can be sipped whenever the woman requires it. Camomile tea can also be drunk, perhaps with ginger root added to enhance the effects.

Price (1993, p.231) recommends petitgrain essential oil dropped on to the pillow to enable the woman to inhale the vapours overnight in preparation for the morning. She also suggests melissa tea made from the fresh herbs.

Labouring women often vomit owing to raised adrenaline levels, stress and hypoglycaemia. Several antiemetic essential oils can be administered to make them feel refreshed and uplifted. Nutmeg oil in low proportions is antiemetic and is thought to have an oestrogenic action, thus strengthening contractions. A flask of hot camomile tea could be made in advance to deal with nausea if it arises, or ice cubes of camomile tea can be sucked throughout labour.

If a newborn baby vomits, the cause must obviously be sought, but in the early days it may be due to ingestion of mucus and fluid at delivery. One of the gentlest essential oils for children is camomile, which is effective as a relaxant, an antispasmodic in cases of colic and an antiemetic. The baby could be bathed in water to which a 1% blend of camomile has been added, or receive an abdominal massage (clockwise) with the same blend. This is a non-invasive means of evacuating ingested amniotic fluid, rather than submitting the baby to a stomach washout. Alternatively, a teaspoon of camomile tea could be administered orally. Mandarin may have similar effects.

An unsuccessful case

Rosemary was admitted to the antenatal ward at six and a half weeks of pregnancy with 'hyperemesis gravidarum' – persistent nausea and vomiting two or three times a day. Conventional antiemetics failed to stop the vomiting and Rosemary seemed unable to eat anything without regurgitation, causing her to avoid eating.

She was given acupressure bands to wear on her wrists at the Pericardium 6 point. Camomile tea with the addition of honey and ginger root was suggested and she was advised to eat grapefruit. Rosemary declined reflexology at this time, preferring not to be 'messed about with'.

Three days after admission Rosemary required an intravenous infusion to replace lost fluid; the wrist bands had been left on but had been moved when the cannula was sited and, needless to say, Rosemary felt that they had been ineffective.

Over the next 2 weeks the complementary therapy midwife visited Rosemary several times to check on her progress and to offer reflexology and/or aromatherapy; finally, in desperation, she agreed to a foot massage incorporating reflexology and using some of the citrus essential oils. This certainly helped her to relax but Rosemary was still not eating and continued to vomit once or twice a day. The consultant decided to commence parenteral nutrition to provide vital nutrients, but agreed with the midwife that, when this was discontinued, homoeopathic remedies could be offered; these were also unsuccessful.

There did, however, appear to be psychological factors contributing to Rosemary's condition. She enjoyed the attention she received from the complementary therapist – to such an extent that eventually it was deemed to be detrimental to her recovery.

Rosemary went home after 3 weeks but, despite several readmissions, no real resolution of the sickness occurred until delivery.

Oedema

Oedema occurs in approximately 50% of all pregnant women towards term, more commonly at the end of the day, and is sometimes worse in the first few days of the puerperium while the kidneys struggle to cope with autolysis and consequent increased diuresis as the mother's body returns to the non-pregnant state. Bimanual upwards massage of the ankles

Fig. 7.13. *Bimanual massage of the legs can be effective in reducing oedema. (See also Plate 8.)*

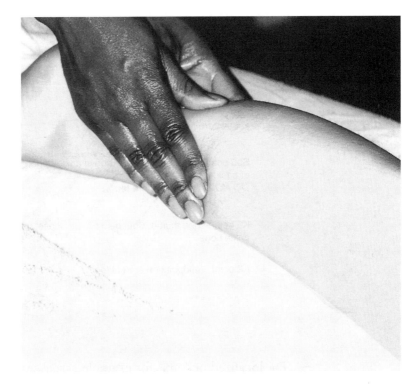

and lower legs will help to relieve excess fluid, and can be very relaxing. This could be demonstrated to the expectant mother by the midwife in the antenatal clinic, who could then ask someone at home to perform it for her. If the mother has bare legs, lubricant will be needed to avoid skin to skin friction, but this does not necessarily have to be a massage oil; talcum powder or soap and water are equally as effective. If the mother is wearing tights, the massage can be carried out without any lubricant as the material will allow the hands to glide freely over the legs (Fig. 7.13).

Oedematous feet in the puerperium can cause the mother both physical and emotional distress, but some gentle massage of the dorsum of each foot, working from the toes towards the ankles, may disperse some of the fluid and give temporary relief. Likewise, finger oedema may be reduced by firm massage of each finger from the nail towards the hand and wrist, and, once demonstrated, the mother could do this for herself.

Shiatsu to the K2 point, on the middle of the arch of the foot, and K6, one thumb's width below the inside of the ankle bone (Fig. 7.14) can also be useful in alleviating ankle oedema, while a general reflexology treatment is relaxing and aids circulation, thereby indirectly easing the oedema.

Essential oils that stimulate the circulation, such as cypress, juniper berry, geranium, lemon, rosemary, patchouli, lavender or ginger, may help. Two of the most effective circulatory stimulants are onion and garlic, but use of the essential oils may be rejected on account of the odours, so these can be added to the diet.

Fig. 7.14. *Shiatsu points for reducing oedema.*

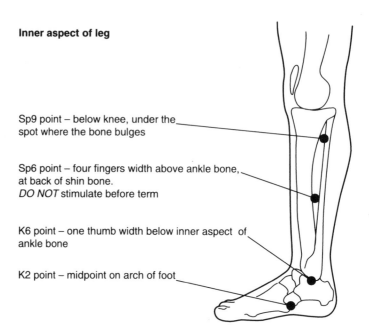

Inner aspect of leg

Sp9 point – below knee, under the spot where the bone bulges

Sp6 point – four fingers width above ankle bone, at back of shin bone.
DO NOT stimulate before term

K6 point – one thumb width below inner aspect of ankle bone

K2 point – midpoint on arch of foot

For localized oedema, for example carpal tunnel syndrome, a compress of juniper berry and/or cypress oils combined with exercise may reduce the intensity of the discomfort; shiatsu on the P6 and P7 points of the inner aspect of the forearm, and TW5 and TW4 on the corresponding parts of the outer arm can be self-administered (Fig. 7.15), or simple hand massage may be used (Fig. 7.13 and Plate 8). Reflex zone therapy has also been found by the author to be particularly effective in easing carpal tunnel syndrome.

Pain relief in labour

Pain is a normal physiological component of labour, caused by the contraction and retraction of the uterine myometrium, but may be exacerbated by psychological, biological, sociocultural and economic factors (Walding 1991). Pain-free labour is considered to be abnormal, as it usually occurs in precipitate labours of multiparous women, which physically and emotionally does not give the woman time to adapt to the impending change from being pregnant to becoming a mother. Much can be done to reduce the intensity of the woman's pain by preparing her antenatally, educating and informing her about the process of labour, facilitating and empowering her to take control of her own labour experience and allaying her fears and anxieties.

Pain can be relieved by stimulating the natural opiate analgesics in the brain, the encephalins and endorphins, either physiologically or chemically, through the use of natural or synthetic pharmacological substances (see Telfer 1997 for more detailed information on conventional methods of pain relief in labour).

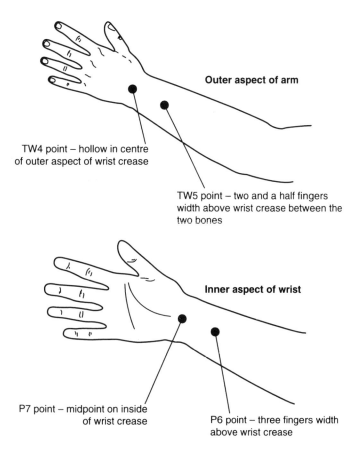

Fig. 7.15. *Shiatsu points to relieve carpal tunnel syndrome.*

Outer aspect of arm

TW4 point – hollow in centre of outer aspect of wrist crease

TW5 point – two and a half fingers width above wrist crease between the two bones

Inner aspect of wrist

P7 point – midpoint on inside of wrist crease

P6 point – three fingers width above wrist crease

Aromatherapy, massage, reflexology and shiatsu offer a range of strategies for alleviating pain and discomfort in labour, although overall care of the mother must remain the responsibility of the midwife. Complementary practitioners who are privileged to assist women in labour *must* be guided by the midwife as to the process and progress of labour, and be prepared to step back from direct care in the event of abnormalities occurring. However, it must also be stressed that the presence of a familiar aromatherapist who can act as a labour companion is invaluable, especially when in many hospital delivery suites midwives have to care for several women simultaneously.

Pain relief in labour may be obtained by using massage, with or without essential oils, especially gentle abdominal effleurage in a clockwise direction. This will serve to lessen the perception of pain as the touch impulses reach the brain before the pain impulses. Labouring women often appreciate neck and shoulder massage to loosen tense muscles. This may be accompanied by gradual pressure being applied to the GB21 shiatsu point on the shoulders (Fig. 7.10).

Foot massage with reflexology can be performed for relaxation and pain relief using brisk massage to the heels and stimulation of the pelvic lymphatic zones across the tops of the ankles (Fig. 7.16). The midwife can suggest that the mother carries out 'wrist wringing' (the equivalent pelvic lymphatic zones on the hands) for 5 min every hour to ease pelvic congestion (Fig. 7.17), together with acupressure to the LI4 point on the hand. Shiatsu to the points in the lumbosacral area (GB27–GB34) is simple and effective, and could be taught to partners (Fig. 7.10).

Essential oils can be a powerful aid to reducing pain intensity in labour, as the chemical constituents and the method of administration will work synergistically. Adding the oils to a base oil for massage incorporates the pharmacological component of the essential oils yet also assists in relaxing the mother, providing her with the 'personal touch', although the practitioner must recognize whether or not the mother wishes to be touched in labour. The oils can be massaged into the feet, abdomen, back and shoulders, depending on the location and intensity of pain and discomfort. Adding the oils to water in the bath or in a foot bath enhances the pain-relieving effects of hydrotherapy (see Garland 2000 for discussion on the benefits and precautions of using water in labour). Essential oils can also be administered via inhalation by putting one or two drops of neat oil onto a cotton wool ball or gauze swab for the mother to sniff when she wishes or by using vaporizers *intermittently* for about 10 minutes out of each hour. Localized compresses can be applied to the suprapubic or sacral areas, a particularly useful method in cases where the fetal occiput is in the posterior position resulting in a long painful labour, often with severe backache. If the mother is becoming very stressed, anxious and

Fig. 7.16. *Reflexology to ease contraction pains.*

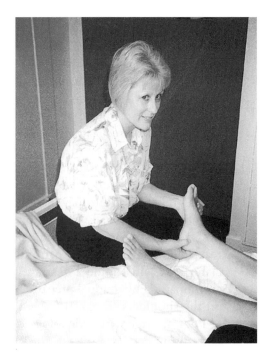

Fig. 7.17. *The mother can be taught 'wrist wringing' to ease pelvic congestion in labour.*

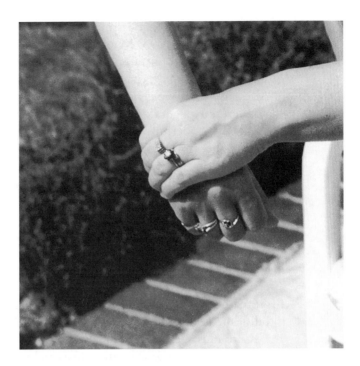

tearful, a single drop of an appropriate essential oil can be rubbed directly onto the solar plexus area beneath the xiphisternum, or to the related reflex zones on the feet, which may help to calm her.

As mentioned above, pain is influenced by a variety of factors, therefore it may be appropriate to select essential oils which, while not necessarily known to be analgesic, may assist in relaxing the mother or easing sickness or other discomforts that will indirectly affect her perception of pain.

Lavender is thought to be effective for the alleviation of both pain and anxiety. Burns & Blamey (1994) used lavender among other oils in their large-scale pilot study and have continued to use it successfully since then (personal communication, 1999). Dale & Cornwell's trial (1994), while focusing on postnatal perineal trauma, found that lavender was more effective in relieving the discomfort than in aiding wound healing. Lavender is known to absorb through the skin (Jager et al 1992) so is probably best administered via massage or in the bath (until the membranes rupture), although Buchbauer et al (1993) also demonstrated its effectiveness when inhaled. Guillemain et al (1989) postulate that lavender may potentiate barbiturates, a factor that may need to be taken into account in relation to drugs used in labour. Lavender and neroli have been shown to have sedative effects (Buchbauer et al 1991, 1993, Imberger et al 1993, Jager et al 1992, Karamat et al 1992), making them useful de-stressing oils for labour. Similarly sandalwood oil is sedative (Okugawa et al 1995). Jasmine has traditionally been used for labouring women and may possess some pain-relieving activity, but is less likely to be relaxing as much of the fairly recent research suggests that jasmine has excitory rather than sedative effects (Imberger et al 1993, Karamat et al 1992, Kikuchi et al 1989). Rose is another essential oil often quoted in standard aromatherapy texts as suitable for labour, and as having an affinity with the female reproductive tract. Although there does not appear to be any supporting research evidence, it is certainly a gentle and pleasant oil to add to a labour blend. Rosewater makes a wonderfully refreshing facial spray to revive the mother during labour and is available commercially (through The Pregnancy Shop, an organization that offers a proportion of its profits for bursaries to enable midwives to train in complementary therapies). Clary sage, frankincense and black pepper may also be used.

Lemongrass has been shown to possess analgesic properties, due to its myrcene content (Lorenzetti et al 1991). Peppermint may be useful for treatment of sickness in labour but may not relieve pain (Nash et al 1986), although more recent trials suggest that it does have pain-relieving properties (Gobel et al 1995). Other essential oils, not currently in popular aromatherapy use in the UK, have also been found to have analgesic capabilities (Almeida et al 1996, Aydin et al 1996, Santos et al 1996, 1997).

Care must be taken with the use of any essential oils during labour, to avoid saturating the air with a heavy, cloying aroma that can be nauseating and which may adversely affect carers as well as the mother and her partner. It is necessary, too, to remember the long-term memory effects of aromas, as demonstrated by Smith et al (1992). Acceptable blends of essential oils for labour, which should be in the lowest possible doses to achieve the desired effect, could include the following, dependent on the mother's needs and wishes:

◆ lavender, clary sage and orange
◆ frankincense, grapefruit and nutmeg
◆ sandalwood and lavender
◆ neroli, orange and rose
◆ lavender and jasmine.

Following delivery, when pain relief such as epidural anaesthesia has caused minor complications, massage, reflexology or shiatsu may be helpful in relieving these, for example stiff neck or back (see Plate 7).

Perineal care

Perineal massage towards term can be performed by the mother if she has a rigid perineum (such as in dancers and horse riders), or when a previous delivery has resulted in considerable scarring of the area. It assists in softening the tissues, increasing elasticity and facilitating the stretching that will occur during delivery, and is thought to reduce the need for episiotomy (Avery & Van Arsdale 1987, Labrecque et al 1994, Mynaugh 1991). It may also help psychologically if the mother is unused to touching this part of her body, and may prepare her for midwifery interventions and care such as vaginal examinations.

The mother can be advised to perform the massage lying on her back in the bath. The thumb is inserted into the introitus with the first two fingers of the hand on the external perineal skin. A gentle massage can be performed, rubbing the thumb and fingers together in an upwards and outwards direction to stretch the perineum. It is not necessary to use any lubricant but if the mother prefers to do this on her bed she may need a little good-quality olive oil.

Some women like to continue perineal massage during labour, and occasionally incorporate clitoral massage which increases the production of endorphins, the brain's natural morphine-like analgesics, and can be very effective in reducing the woman's perception of contraction pain.

In the puerperium, perineal care revolves around easing discomfort, promoting healing and preventing infection. Dale & Cornwell's (1994) trial involved the use of essential oil of lavender in the bath, and although the results in relation to wound healing were not considered statistically significant, there is some evidence that mothers experienced less perineal discomfort between the third and fifth postnatal day. Experience in the author's maternity unit supports this, and mothers have (anecdotally) been found to be more relaxed when using lavender in twice-daily baths for a number of days.

Lavender, having antibacterial properties, is effective in preventing infection, although if an episiotomy wound shows signs of infection the use of tea tree in the bidet is advocated. Camomile, eucalyptus or thyme may also be of use, while geranium or juniper berry oils aid healing, partly due to their astringent vasoconstrictive action.

Placenta, retained

In women who have successfully completed the second stage of labour but in whom the placenta is slower than normal to separate, essential oils can be used to initiate uterine action. Jasmine oil, massaged over the fundus, lavender or clary sage can be used. It may, however, be easier and more effective for the midwife to perform reflexology on the foot zones relating to both the uterus and the pituitary gland to stimulate uterine contraction (Fig. 7.11).

A compress of basil or camomile oil applied suprapubically can relieve 'afterpains', aid involution and encourage any retained products to be expelled.

Preconception care and infertility

Midwives may not often come into contact with women who are planning to conceive, but they may be asked for information regarding the use of aromatherapy for subsequent pregnancies.

As with all drugs, essential oils should be used with caution during the preconception period and in the first trimester of pregnancy, and self-administration should perhaps be discouraged. Aromatherapy can be of value in relaxing couples whose desire to conceive is proving emotionally and physically stressful. Gentle oils such as orange, mandarin, grapefruit, frankincense and ylang ylang could be used in low dilutions for massage or in the bath. Culinary herbs could be added to the diet as a means of obtaining small amounts of the necessary essential oils.

Massage, reflexology or shiatsu relax either the prospective mother or father, and could then be continued into the pregnancy. Experience of this author and other reflex zone therapists in identifying, on the relevant foot zones, when and from which ovary ovulation has occurred, and in tracking the movement of the ovum along the fallopian tube, may indicate a potential use for reflexology in the treatment of infertility. It should theoretically be possible for stimulation of the foot zones related to the pituitary gland and the ovary to trigger ovulation.

Respiratory problems

Pregnant women may suffer coughs, colds and sinus congestion, that appear to be coincidental to the pregnancy. However, in Oriental medicine this is thought to be related to a weakened kidney energy and may occur as a direct response to the pregnant state (Johnson 2000, p. 196). The midwife could refer the mother to a qualified shiatsu practitioner for rebalancing of energy throughout the body. Chronic sinus congestion may be eased by eliminating dairy produce from the diet, as it is known to increase mucus production.

Symptomatic relief can be obtained with aromatherapy. For infectious respiratory conditions such as colds and influenza, essential oils of tea tree, eucalyptus, benzoin, clary sage, frankincense or marjoram can be inhaled and will both ease congestion and loosen mucus and also act as an antibacterial agent, although early research by Boyd & Sheppard (1970) suggested that, for eucalyptus to be effective as a decongestant and mucolytic, the dose would have to be so high as to cause local dermal toxicity. Lavender can be effective when the mother has an accompanying headache, but only during the last trimester. The oils can be massaged into the upper back, using effleurage and some percussion techniques to aid mucus drainage. Adding garlic to the diet will fight any infection, or teas made from basil or camomile can be suggested.

Conventional treatment for bronchitis may be enhanced by using inhalations of lavender or mint (Shubina et al 1990).

Reflex zone therapy to the thoracic and head zones on the feet may assist expectoration of mucus and relieve headache, respectively. Acupressure to the B2, LI20 and St3 points can ease sinus congestion, headache, tired eyes and other cold symptoms (Fig. 7.18).

Sexual difficulties

Many expectant and newly delivered women experience a variety of emotional and physical symptoms that can adversely affect libido and physical comfort during sex. The more serious problems may require referral to an appropriate counsellor, but some difficulties can be resolved with aromatherapy.

Psychological and emotional factors may be helped by offering essential oil massages and/or baths using blends containing aphrodisiac ylang ylang, neroli and sandalwood during pregnancy, plus rose, patchouli, clary

Fig. 7.18. Shiatsu points for sinus congestion.

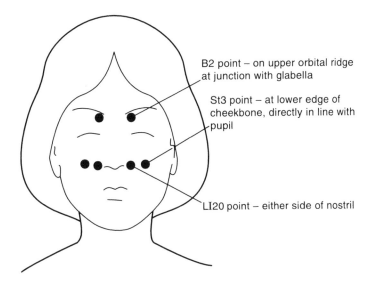

B2 point – on upper orbital ridge at junction with glabella

St3 point – at lower edge of cheekbone, directly in line with pupil

LI20 point – either side of nostril

sage and jasmine in the puerperium. These may help to relax the woman (and her partner), and may work indirectly on the libido. Black pepper and cardamom may have a directly stimulating effect and can be of use when fatigue is a predisposing factor, but they should be administered with caution only as a temporary measure.

If physical factors are contributing to sexual difficulties, the appropriate essential oils can be applied to deal with a sore perineum, thrush, leucorrhoea, etc.

Skin care

During the childbearing year some women find their skin becomes dehydrated, while others experience oiliness in the form of acne and skin eruptions. Many mothers develop striae gravidarum, usually as full term approaches. A few, especially brunettes and darker-skinned women, are bothered by excess melanin production, which results not only in pigmentation of the linea alba, but also facial chloasma. Aromatherapy has several remedies to offer for skin care; indeed, many people think that aromatherapy is only concerned with beauty care.

Dry skin may be helped by using gentle essential oils such as orange, neroli or rose in a base oil enriched with a small amount of avocado and wheatgerm oils. Apricot kernel or peach kernel are good base oils for facial massage. The mother can be advised to massage the oils into the skin very gently to avoid further damage. In early pregnancy the base oil can be used on its own.

The high levels of circulating hormones can, in some women, have much the same effect as at the time of puberty, resulting in oily skin or even acne. Astringent and antibacterial essential oils are useful in these cases, including bergamot, cypress, lemon and sandalwood, and are best administered via a facial sauna rather than as a massage oil. Tea tree oil can be added to the blend if there are numerous spots; one drop can be applied neat to an isolated eruption, or a water-based spray can be applied over the whole area.

There is no evidence to indicate that application of any oil, lotion or cream can prevent striae gravidarum from developing, despite the plethora of proprietary products claiming to do so. If a mother wishes to apply aromatherapy oils to her abdomen to moisturize the outer skin, the most suitable are neroli and mandarin, possibly used in rotation with bergamot and rosewood. They can be applied after 16 weeks, in a base oil of soya, avocado and wheatgerm.

Chloasma, unfortunately, is unlikely to respond to treatment with aromatherapy oils, although lemon essential oil acts as a mild bleaching agent, as may benzoin. However, as daily use over a protracted period of time may be needed for the oil to take effect, the value of aromatherapy in reducing gestational chloasma is limited.

Eczema responds well to essential oils of lavender and camomile, and babies who develop the condition could be treated by adding two drops of essential oil to the bathwater, using camomile for 1 week, lavender for 1 week with a 1-week interval between. It must be recognized, however, that in many cases this may treat the symptoms but not the cause of the eczema.

Stress and anxiety

Anxiety and stress are common during pregnancy and childbearing for a number of reasons, including fear of the unknown, concerns about the fetus/baby and lack of confidence. Obviously aromatherapy cannot take the place of sensitive midwifery care, talking and counselling. In many respects, however, this is one condition where aromatherapy comes into its own, and indeed is most likely to be perceived as acceptable by sceptical colleagues. There are several essential oils that can be used to combat stress, although many are contraindicated during pregnancy. If there is any doubt regarding the safety of an essential oil, a simple massage – of feet, shoulders or back – using base oil alone is extremely relaxing.

Sedative and calming oils, including benzoin, bergamot, frankincense, geranium, mandarin, neroli, petitgrain, sandalwood and ylang ylang, are suitable for use in pregnancy. Other oils that can be administered near term, during labour or after delivery include camomile, clary sage, cypress, geranium, juniper berry, lavender, marjoram, melissa, patchouli and rose.

There are a few other oils that are classified as sedative, such as cedarwood, celery, linden blossom, sage, verbena and vetivert, but these are not suitable for use in maternity care.

The most relaxing method of application may be in a massage, but adding a blend to the bathwater or inhaling the aromas from a vaporizer will save time; respiratory tract administration is thought to have a direct effect upon the limbic system and on mood (Buchbauer et al 1991, 1993). If the anxiety is causing physical symptoms, oils can be selected specifically to relieve them. These would include (depending on the gestation) bergamot or marjoram for muscle tension, mandarin or neroli for stomach upsets, ylang ylang or lavender for raised blood pressure, lavender for headaches, and ylang ylang or camomile for insomnia. As a universal 'standby' that can be used from the second trimester in small doses, in labour, in the puerperium and for the neonate, the optimum essential oil must be mandarin, particularly when given in a massage. However, administration should not be continuous for more than 3 weeks, and is best alternated with other oils to avoid allergy or irritation developing.

Urinary tract problems

Frequency of micturition is a physiological symptom of pregnancy caused mainly by the pressure of the enlarging uterus on the bladder during the first trimester and by the engaging fetal head towards term, although many women experience frequency and urgency to micturate throughout pregnancy. Poor pelvic floor control will add to this and lead to stress incontinence.

Dilation of the ureters under the influence of progesterone results in a tendency to stasis of urine and a predisposition towards urinary tract infection, with some women developing asymptomatic bacteriuria and others experiencing cystitis. It is important that urinary tract infections are diagnosed and treated as unresolved infection can lead to pyelonephritis, owing to the gestational changes in renal filtration and function, or may precipitate preterm labour.

Essential oils may be used prophylactically against urinary tract infection by adding them to the bathwater or as a localized douche or swabbing solution around the external meatus of the urethra. Suprapubic compresses of warm water with essential oils may be effective in administering antibacterial aromatherapy and as a means of relieving low abdominal pain; similarly compresses applied to the sacral and hip areas may alleviate or reduce kidney pain. Any of the antibacterial essential oils could be used, especially tea tree. Sandalwood and camomile are quoted in some aromatherapy texts as having an affinity with the urinary tract, while drinking camomile tea may act as a urinary cleanser. Camomile oil may be effective in treating infection of the urinary tract through its anti-inflammatory action (Tubaro et al 1984), probably due to the α-bisabolol content (Carle & Gomaa 1992) although Safayhi et al (1994) attribute the anti-inflammatory and other effects of camomile to the chamazulene produced in the extraction of the essential oil from the plant.

Retention of urine may be a problem postnatally, most commonly due to localized oedema as a result of a traumatic delivery, or less frequently due to neurogenic damage. Retention of urine can occur also at approximately 16–20 weeks of pregnancy where the mother has a retroverted uterus that fails to antevert spontaneously. In these cases reflex zone therapy offers a relatively simple means of stimulating micturition, although care should be taken to ensure the cause of the retention is understood so that the most appropriate reflexology technique can be used. Some essential oils are thought to stimulate diuresis (Stanic & Samarzija 1993) although 'white-headed' camomile oil has been shown to have an antidiuretic action (Rossi et al 1988).

Sally had developed antenatal retention of urine at 16 weeks which, although not confirmed by ultrasound investigation, was deemed to be due to a retroverted gravid uterus. The complementary therapy midwife was asked to see her at 20 weeks' gestation, by which time Sally had a self-retaining catheter in situ (although she was still an outpatient). The midwife performed reflex zone therapy, and on examination was astounded to feel, on the relevant part of Sally's feet, that the zone for the uterus was further back on the heel than would normally be felt. This seemed to indicate that the assumed diagnosis of retroversion was correct.

The midwife carried out one full session of reflex zone therapy, after which Sally spontaneously passed 400 ml urine. One might consider that, at 20 weeks' gestation, the situation may have resolved itself anyway, but it is interesting that spontaneous micturition occurred shortly after the first treatment. The catheter was removed and was not needed again. Sally chose to continue to receive reflex zone therapy regularly and was able to enjoy her pregnancy to the full. Following a normal delivery of a large boy, she was unable to pass urine spontaneously for 18 hours, but reflex zone therapy was again successful.

Vaginal infections   Although many women experience normal increased vaginal discharge (leucorrhoea) as a result of excess cervical mucus and vaginal transudate due to increased vascularity, a few develop infections in the reproductive tract as a result of the altered pH and changes in vaginal flora. These not only cause irritation, sometimes offensive discharge and discomfort, but also place the fetus at risk of acquiring the infection on its journey down the birth canal. The commonest vaginal infections are due to the yeast-like fungus, *Candida albicans* (thrush), bacterial *Chlamydia*, protozoal *Trichomonas*, viral genital herpes and, less commonly, syphilis, caused by a spirochaete and bacterial gonorrhoea. Some of these may be present prior to conception or manifest themselves during pregnancy.

Severe infections will, of course, require the appropriate pharmaceutical treatment, but essential oils may be used as an alternative for minor cases or as an enhancement to drug therapy. Essential oils may be used successfully for many bacterial and fungal infections (see also Bacterial infections, p. 75), the oil of choice being tea tree (*Melaleuca alternifolia*), either as a vaginal douche or tampon – soaked intravaginal application or added to the bathwater in which the woman can sit. The dilution should be kept to 1% as there have been several reports of contact dermatitis from tea tree (De Groot & Weyland 1992, 1993, Knight & Hausen 1994) and the already-irritated and delicate mucosa of the vagina may be extra sensitive at this time, although in Belaiche's treatment (1985a) of 28 women using tea tree pessaries, only one discontinued due to irritation. Tea tree oil pessaries are available in health stores for self-administration; indeed one of the earlier reported successes was of a pregnant woman who refused conventional treatment for candidal infection, preferring instead to use pessaries (Department of Genito-urinary Medicine 1991). Carson & Riley (1994) in Australia suggest that *Melaleuca alternifolia* may have a vital role to play in the treatment of candidiasis, especially in the light of the limited range of topical antifungal agents. Tea tree oil has also been used to treat trichomonal infection (Pena 1962) and may be effective against herpes, HIV infection and genital warts.

Melissa was found to be more effective than either lavender or rosemary oil against *Candida* (Larrondo & Calvo 1991), while juniper berry oil may also be antifungal (Mishra & Chauhan 1984). *Eucalyptus maidenii* has similar effects (Gundidza et al 1993). Twenty one eucalyptus oils were tested against several microbes, including *Candida*, and *Eucalyptus citriodora* was shown to be the most effective inhibitor (Hajji & Fkih-Tetouani 1993, Zakarya et al 1993). New Zealand kanuka oil has proved to be similar to tea tree in its antimicrobial activity (Cooke & Cooke 1991). Interestingly, Abdel Wahab et al (1987) found that frankincense oil was effective against a range of organisms *except Candida* and *Pseudomonas*.

Valnet's collation (1982) of 268 clinical cases of infection showed the best success rate with marjoram (88%) compared with several other oils. Research by Galal et al (1973) also compared a range of essential oils, with lavender and lemon having only minor fungistatic activity, and patchouli being particularly recommended for its effect on yeast infections. Conversely, Yang et al (1996) found resistance of *Candida albicans* to certain types of patchouli. Viollon et al (1996) investigated the effects of 30 essential oils on non-pathogenic and pathogenic vaginal flora, and found that santalol adversely affected *Neisseria gonorrhoea*, while cinnamon, geranium and mint oils as well as certain of their constituents, were antifungal against *Candida albicans*. Rosemary essential oil will also inhibit *Candida* (Domokos et al 1997, Soliman et al 1994, Steinmetz et al 1987) and both cardamom and cumin oils may have similar actions, probably due to the terpinyl acetate (ester) and linalool (alcohol) content of the former and cumaldehyde (aldehyde) in the latter (Badei 1992, Singh & Upadhyay 1991), although Farag et al (1989) found cumin not to act on Gram-negative bacteria. The fungitoxic action of *Citrus sinensis* (sweet orange) oil is thought to be due to the limonene content, although this constituent appears to need the synergistic effect within the whole oil as it is less effective in isolation (Singh et al 1993), an important consideration when selecting appropriate essential oils. Recent research by Suresh et al (1995,

1997) indicates that santolina oil may have strong anticandidal activity and compares favourably with standard pharmaceutical antifungal preparations. Oregano has also been found to inhibit *Candida*; this action is thought to be due to the carvacrol content (Juven et al 1994, Stiles et al 1995).

Cultures of *Trichomonas* were exposed to 26 essential oils by Viollon et al (1996). It was found that cinnamon, vetiver and sandalwood were strongly effective, followed by ylang ylang, juniper berry and lemongrass, while lavender and cajeput had no effect; of the isolated constituents, thymol was shown to have the best antitrichomonal activity.

Varicosities

Varicose veins of the legs are usually temporary, developing in pregnancy as a result of the action of progesterone in relaxing the smooth walls of the blood vessels, and exacerbated by pressure from increasing abdominal weight. Complete resolution will not be achieved until after delivery, but essential oil of cypress in the bathwater may assist in toning the circulation and reducing the throbbing pain that often accompanies varicose veins. Massage directly over varicosed areas is contraindicated, but gently gliding the hands over the leg will give an impression of 'completeness', especially during a full body massage.

Similarly, if a mother suffers from vulval varicosities, cypress, juniper berry or lavender oil added to a bidet are astringent and help to soothe the discomfort.

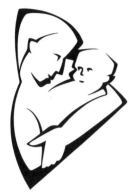

Chapter 8   # Directory of Oils for Use in Maternity Care

Comprehensive information about individual essential oils can be found in many aromatherapy textbooks, and readers are referred to the list of Further reading in the References section for those recommended by the author, although this list is by no means exhaustive. Readers should be mindful of the many unsubstantiated claims for essential oils, and should endeavour always, where possible, to refer to contemporary validated research findings.

However, for ease of learning for those new to the subject of aromatherapy, a selection of essential oils suitable for use with pregnant, labouring and puerperal women and their newborn babies is included here, with emphasis on aspects of particular relevance to the client group. There is some repetition between this chapter and the previous one, but this should enable a cross-referencing system to be used, so that readers can either refer to a specific essential oil or find information on oils most suited to the treatment of different conditions.

Each essential oil is identified by its Latin name; the main chemical constituents, and the uses and contraindications or dangers pertinent to maternity care are discussed.

The 30 essential oils outlined here are:

- Basil
- Benzoin
- Bergamot
- Black pepper
- Camomile
- Clary sage
- Eucalyptus
- Frankincense
- Geranium
- Ginger
- Grapefruit
- Jasmine
- Juniper berry
- Lavender
- Lemon
- Lemongrass
- Lime
- Mandarin

- Marjoram
- Neroli
- Nutmeg
- Orange
- Patchouli
- Petitgrain

- Rose
- Rosemary
- Rosewood
- Sandalwood
- Tea tree
- Ylang ylang

Basil – *Ocimum basilicum* (Labiatae family)

There are many different types of basil oil available but the one normally used in aromatherapy has a spicy aroma, derived by steam distillation from the flowers and leaves.

Chemical constituents   Basil oil is very stimulating, even in small doses, due to the proportion of esters (about 8% according to Price 1993, p. 54) and the monoterpenes limonene and pinene. The presence of the ketone, camphor, not only adds to the stimulant effect but is also an emmenagogue, so basil is *contraindicated in pregnancy*. However, the monoterpenes, ketones and a high level of phenols mean that basil has analgesic properties and can be of help in low dilutions in labour and the puerperium.

The amount of phenols is reputed to be as high as 87% (Tisserand & Balacs 1995, p. 190), which makes the essential oil an effective antiseptic. One of the principal phenols is estragole or methyl chavicol, which has been thought to be carcinogenic in high doses. Consequently, Tisserand & Balacs (1995, p. 203) suggest that only basil varieties with low (i.e. below 5%) methyl chavicol concentrations should be used in clinical aromatherapy. Phenols, together with the alcohols, fenchol, linalol and citronellol and the oxide 1,8-cineole, have decongestant and expectorant effects so that basil can be used for inhalations in the event of chest infection, perhaps after a Caesarean section. Women who suffer respiratory tract congestion and sinus problems in pregnancy could make basil tea from the leaves, thus ensuring a weaker solution, and inhale the vapours. The antifungal properties of *Ocimum basilicum* have also been demonstrated (Dube et al 1989), although Ndounga & Ouamba (1997) found only moderate antimicrobial activity. Various strains of *Ocimum* essential oils are also larvicidal and mosquito-repellant (Bhatnagae et al 1993, Chokechaijaroenporn et al 1994). 1993).

Basil is effective for headache and migraine, although there are other, safer oils which can be used in pregnancy for this complaint.

The antispasmodic action of basil as a result of the esters and phenols make it a useful oil for digestive complaints. The oestrogenic effects mean that it can aid placental separation in the third stage of labour and ease 'after pains' and breast engorgement in the early puerperium, as well as helping in cases of dysmenorrhoea and the menopause. It is thought to have a possible value in treating hormonally related infertility. Indeed, the stimulation of blood flow and the hormonal influence of basil, coupled

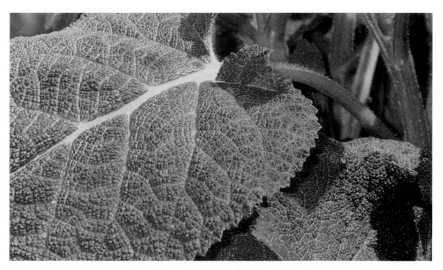

Plate 1 *Salvia sclarea* (clary sage).

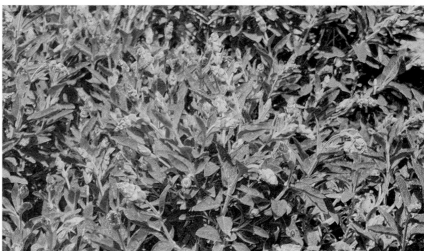

Plate 2 *Salvia officinalis* (sage). *Note the difference between the common garden sage and clary sage.*

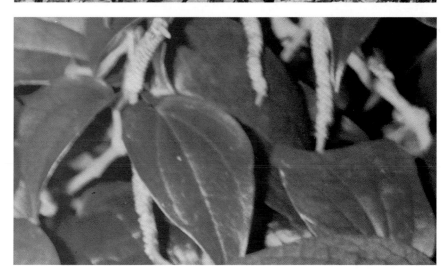

Plate 3 *Piper nigrum* (black pepper).

Plate 4 *Pelargonium officinalis* Graveolens (geranium).

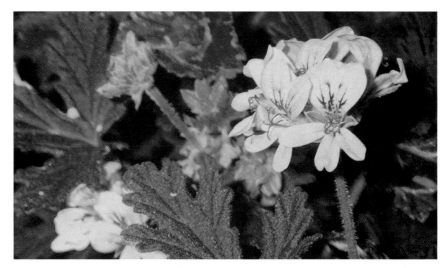

Plate 5 *Origanum vulgare* (marjoram).

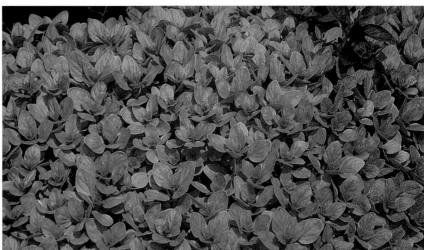

Plate 6 *Rosmarinus officinalis* (rosemary).

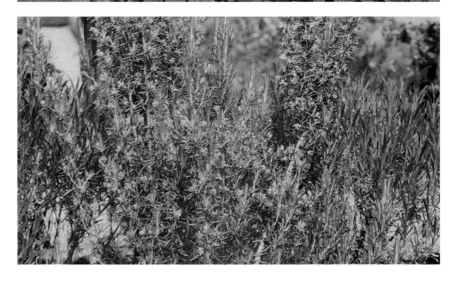

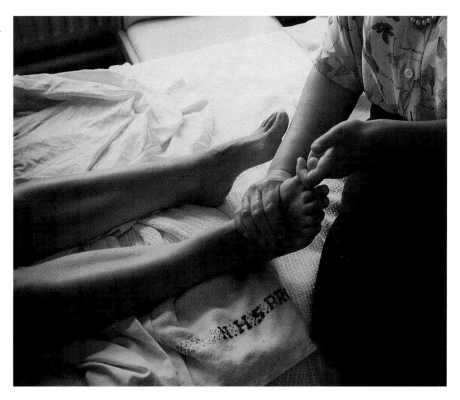

Plate 7 Woman receiving reflex zone therapy for stiff neck following epidural anaesthesia.

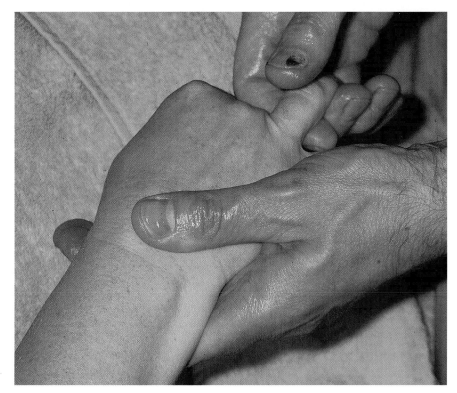

Plate 8 Woman receiving hand massage to reduce oedematous fingers.

with the effect on mental fatigue, make this a suitable oil to combine with others for massage in the early postnatal days.

Dangers Basil is *contraindicated in pregnancy* because it is a stimulant and an emmenagogue, but more particularly because of the methyl chavicol. Care should be taken when purchasing basil oil to ensure that the methyl chavicol content is below 5%. Methyl chavicol can cause skin irritation to those with sensitive skin; there has also been speculation about potential carcinogenic effects of basil, although Aruna & Sivaramakrishnan (1996) suggest that the ability of basil oil to increase the activity of glutathione *S*-transferase, a carcinogen–detoxifying enzyme, may point to its potential as an anticarcinogen. High concentrations can reverse the generally stimulating effect and cause the recipient to become soporific. Basil oil may be mildly toxic when administered orally so is best avoided by mouth.

Blends Basil will blend well with bergamot, black pepper, clary sage, frankincense, geranium, grapefruit, lavender, lemongrass, mandarin, marjoram, neroli, rosemary, sandalwood and tangerine.

Benzoin – *Styrax benzoin* (Styracea family)

Benzoin comes from the eastern areas of Thailand and Java, and the resin is obtained from the bark of the tree. Solvent extraction (often with wood alcohol) is used to release the aromatic material from the resin. The aroma is pleasant and rather like vanilla.

Chemical constituents Benzoin has an impact on the kidneys, stimulating renal output and, with its antiseptic property resulting from the aldehydes benzoic aldehyde and vanillin (which give it the characteristic aroma), may be of use in cystitis. Aldehydes can also be hypotensive in action. It is useful for treating colic, flatulence and constipation (in the mother), owing to the antispasmodic action of the ester benzyl benzoate, and may help to control blood sugar levels. Coelho-de-Souza et al (1997) found that the estragole content of another essential oil, *Croton zehntneri*, was responsible for an antispasmodic effect on guinea pig ileum, although it was noted that the whole essential oil was more effective than the isolated constituent, prompting the caution of attributing properties of essential oils to individual constituents.

Although benzoin is uplifting and stimulating, it is not an emmenagogue, so unlike basil could safely be used in low dilutions from mid-pregnancy, although the therapeutic effects of benzoin can be found in other oils which have been more frequently used on pregnant women. Its action on the respiratory tract, particularly in stimulating mucus flow, results in benzoin being useful as an inhalation for sinusitis, bronchitis, colds and coughs, and sore throats.

Benzoin is popularly known as Friar's Balsam for healing skin wounds, especially where there is dermatitis. It is theoretically possible that chloasma may be reduced if benzoin is added to a skin toner, although this would probably require daily use over a period of time, a practice which is contraindicated in aromatherapy generally. The wound-healing and anti-inflammatory effects are probably due to the presence of acids – benzoic and cinnamic. However, cases of sensitivity to benzoin dressings have been reported (Cullen et al 1974, James et al 1984, Lesesne 1992, Mann 1982, Rademaker & Kirby 1987, Tripathi et al 1990).

Stress, tension and anxiety can be calmed by using benzoin in a massage blend as it has a sedative effect and assists in easing worries and improving self-confidence; this may be of help in the postnatal period for some mothers.

Dangers If used to excess benzoin may cause drowsiness; in some people it may also cause allergic skin reactions (see above).

Blends Benzoin can be blended with bergamot, camomile, eucalyptus, frankincense, juniper berry, lavender, lemon, mandarin, orange, neroli, petitgrain, rose and sandalwood.

Bergamot – *Citrus bergamia* (Rutaceae family)

Essential oil of bergamot is obtained by expression of the rind of the fruit from the tree, which is native to Italy. The aroma is mainly orange and lemon, and the oil is emerald green in colour.

Chemical constituents The proportion of alcohols, including linalol, nerol and geraniol, and the aldehyde citral mean that bergamot has antiseptic properties coupled with an affinity for the urogenital tract, and provides a safe and effective means of treating cystitis and urinary tract infection throughout the reproductive year. It can relieve gastrointestinal complaints for which an antispasmodic is needed such as indigestion, colic and flatulence, as there are up to 50% esters (Ryman 1991, p. 53), including linalyl acetate, in bergamot oil. It is also thought to stimulate the appetite.

Monoterpenes (limonene, pinene and camphene), as well as the esters, give bergamot its antiseptic, antibacterial, antiviral and antifungal characteristics. Respiratory tract infections respond well to inhalations of bergamot oil, as do certain viral infections such as herpes simplex and varicella because of the large amount of the aldehyde citral. Women who suffer from acne during pregnancy may find a facial sauna using bergamot will help to alleviate the condition. Citral is also responsible for acting as a hypotensive agent, as are the coumarins, mainly in the form of bergapten. Coumarins can have an anticoagulant effect and, although the proportion of these is small, it may be wise to use low dilutions towards term when the mother's own clotting mechanisms adapt to the impending labour. Bergamottine has also been found to have antianginal and antiarrhythmic properties (Occhiutto & Circosta 1996a, 1996b).

Bergamot may help to tone the uterus and can be a good oil to use in labour, especially as it is also a very calming yet uplifting oil, possibly owing to its action on the sympathetic nervous system. It is antispasmodic and anti-inflammatory owing to the presence of esters, while camphene, limonene and pinene (terpenes) are analgesic. Occhiuto et al (1995) also found the non-volatile residue from the *Citrus bergamia* essential oil to have central nervous system effects, suggesting it may have sedative, anti-convulsant and analgesic properties.

Dangers   The presence of a 0.44% concentration of the furocoumarins bergapten and bergamottine, which stimulate melanin production, means that this essential oil should be used with care. Zaynoun et al (1977) found bergapten to be the only significant phototoxic agent, with the degree of phototoxicity correlating with the concentration of bergapten. This is particularly important when there is bright sunlight, for excessive and irregular discoloration of exposed skin can occur; these areas of the body may possibly degenerate at a later stage and lead to early skin cancer. Reported cases in the 1970s (Meyer 1970) of skin reactions to tanning agents containing bergamot, severe enough to require admission to a burns unit, eventually led to the oil being omitted from suntanning creams and lotions. Ryman (1991, p. 54) suggests that it should rarely be used as a massage oil, although other authorities state that it may be used in a 1–2% dilution (International School of Aromatherapy 1993, p. 75), while Price (1993, p. 54) argues that it is fully absorbed into the bloodstream within an hour, after which time the phototoxicity is negated. However, the raised melanocytic hormone levels during pregnancy emphasize the need for caution when using bergamot, as irregular patches of pigmentation may develop if the skin is exposed to the sun immediately after using high dilutions of the oil. Tisserand & Balacs (1995, p. 121) cite the IFRA recommendation to keep bergamot oil to below 0.4% dilution if it is to be applied to areas of skin exposed to sunshine.

In addition the high citral content could potentially impair reproductive performance (Toaff et al 1979).

Blends   Bergamot essential oil has a gentle aroma that blends well with basil, benzoin, black pepper, camomile, clary sage, eucalyptus, geranium, grapefruit, jasmine, juniper berry, lavender, lemon, mandarin, marjoram, neroli, orange, patchouli, petitgrain, rose, tangerine and ylang ylang.

Black pepper –
Piper nigrum
(Piperaceae family)

Essential oil of black pepper is distilled from the fruit and seeds of the tree and, as might be expected, has a spicy peppery aroma, which appeals to men but which can also add interest to a more feminine blend (Plate 3).

Chemical constituents   The high concentration of monoterpenes (camphene, farnesene, limonene, myrcene, pinene, sabinene and thujene) and sesquiterpenes (caryophyllene) makes black pepper an excellent analgesic, and its vasodilatory effects make it valuable in cases of muscular aches, pains and stiffness. It is beneficial both before and after strenuous physical activity, and lends itself to pain relief in labour; it is also stimulating and seems to give mental stamina which could help a woman having a long, slow first stage. (It is interesting to note that it may be beneficial in reducing smoking withdrawal symptoms (Rose & Behm 1994).)

Alcohols in the form of linalol and pinocarvol give black pepper a warming action which improves the circulation, making it beneficial for bruising. The oil could be applied postnatally in a massage to the buttocks where forceps delivery has resulted in excessive trauma. Despite its rubefacient characteristic, black pepper can also be used in small doses, almost in a homoeopathic way, to reduce pyrexia. The essential oil may increase the production of red blood cells, which could be valuable in cases of anaemia.

Black pepper contains phenols – carvocrol, eugenol, safrole and myristicin – which affect the digestive system. Its laxative properties make it a useful aid to increasing peristalsis and reducing flatulence. It is thought to help the digestion of proteins and the excretion of toxins, leading to weight loss, so it may appeal to women for use towards the end of the puerperium. The oil has strong diuretic properties but should not be used directly for this purpose as overdosing could precipitate excessive renal stimulation; low doses are advised during pregnancy to avoid potential damage to kidney function.

Dangers   The above-mentioned diuretic effect needs to be taken into consideration when using black pepper in pregnancy. Very small amounts can be beneficial but care should be taken that it is blended with other oils to reduce the concentration. It is also possible that higher concentrations may lead to skin irritation, so vaporization rather than massage may be the preferred method of administration. Ryman (1991, p. 159) comments on its myristicin content, which, although much lower than the amount in nutmeg or mace oils, may be sufficient to preclude its use during pregnancy (see also Nutmeg).

Blends   Small amounts of black pepper give a blend an interesting spiciness and it mixes well with basil, bergamot, frankincense, geranium, grapefruit, lemon, mandarin, nutmeg, patchouli, rosemary, sandalwood and ylang ylang.

Camomiles – *Matricaria chamomilla* and *Anthemis nobilis* (Compositae family)

There are several different types of camomile essential oil available, each with slightly different, though mainly similar, properties. The commonest camomiles used in aromatherapy are German camomile, *Matricaria chamomilla*, and the purer and more expensive Roman camomile, *Anthemis nobilis*. A Moroccan variety, *Ormenis multicaulis*, is also sometimes used. All camomiles belong to the Compositae family, but it is important to obtain the essential oil from a reputable supplier and to ask for it by its Latin name as the proportion of the chemical constituents varies from one type to another. (This is similar to the need to ask for drugs by their trade name rather than the generic name to ensure the exact composition.)

The two most commonly used camomile essential oils will be considered here: German and Roman camomiles.

Matricaria chamomilla   Despite its name, the plant is no longer grown in Germany for essential oil production, but comes mainly from eastern Europe, particularly Hungary. The essential oil is distilled from the flowers and initially is a bluish colour which gradually alters to a greenish yellow colour. The depth of the blue coloration is dependent on the amount of chamazulene, a constituent that is not present in the flower but develops during the process of extracting the essential oil, and German camomile tends to be deeper blue than Roman as it contains more chamazulene. It is interesting to note that the term *Matricaria* comes from the Latin meaning uterus, and indeed camomile has a long history in folk medicine of being used for gynaecological problems.

Chemical constituents   The presence of the sesquiterpene, azulene, a fatty substance which forms during the production process, together with matricine, results in German camomile's anti-inflammatory and wound-healing properties; it is especially effective in treating skin problems such as eczema. Carle & Gomaa (1992) found that the anti-inflammatory property of *Matricaria* was due, not only to the chamazulene and matricine, but also to apigenin-7-glucoside and α-bisabolol, with the latter being the most effective. Of four chemotypes investigated, only one contained α-bisabolol; it was recommended by the authors that pharmaceutical preparations of camomile (ointment, etc.) should contain the two newly discovered components. This confirmed earlier work by Isaac (1979) and Jakovlev et al (1983). Bisabolol may also have an ulcer-protective action (Szelenyi & Thiemer 1979). The components of various types of camomile oil responsible for its antiphlogistic action continue to be investigated (Miller et al 1996).

Azulene and another sesquiterpene, farnesene, together with the alcohols, farnesol and bisabolol, and the aldehyde, cuminic acid, also contribute to the antiseptic, antibacterial, antifungal and antiviral functions of camomile; Ryman (1991, p. 77) states that camomile may be 120 times more effective than saline in acting as an antiseptic.

Camomile seems to have a particular affinity for the urinary tract, so women with a urinary tract infection or cystitis could drink camomile tea as a urinary cleanser. Using a dilute solution of the tea as an eye cleanser may prevent or treat ophthalmia neonatorum.

Soaked and cooled camomile teabags placed over sore and bleeding nipples can ease discomfort and speed healing, without danger to the infant of accidentally ingesting a harmful substance that might otherwise be applied to heal the nipples. However, two mothers are reported to have developed contact dermatitis of the nipple after applying Kamillosan cream, a popular cream containing essential oil of camomile (McGeorge & Steele 1991). Interestingly, one mother was using a British brand of Kamillosan which contains Roman camomile while the other, in Europe, was using a brand containing German camomile. On the other hand the wound-healing, anti-inflammatory and analgesic properties of *M. chamomilla* have been well documented (Aertgeerts et al 1985, Glowania et al 1987, Nissen et al 1988, Tubaro et al 1984). It can safely be surmised that sitting in a bath to which camomile oil has been added may assist in healing the perineum following delivery, and will help to relax the mother.

Research by Safayhi et al (1994) suggests that the antiphlogistic effects of camomile may be due to the inhibition by chamazulene of the production of leucotrienes, found in patients with various inflammatory diseases.

A small amount of camphor, which is a ketone, means that camomile is an emmenagogue, so use of the essential oil should be *avoided in early pregnancy*, although judicious use in later pregnancy is acceptable and the beneficial effects of camomile's constituents can be obtained by drinking the tea during the first and second trimesters.

Ketones and sesquiterpenes make camomile a good analgesic: teabags placed against the neck over the eustachian tube can ease earache; the essential oil massaged into the back relieves backache, dysmenorrhoea or the pain of contractions and afterpains; headaches may also be helped by using camomile.

Anthemis nobilis Although there are many similarities in the therapeutic properties of *A. nobilis* and *M. chamomilla*, the plants are very different, with *A. nobilis* being shorter, the stems hairier and the white daisy-like flowers larger than those of *M. chamomilla*.

Chemical constituents As with German camomile, the essential oil of *A. nobilis* contains chamazulene (sesquiterpene) and cuminic acid (aldehyde), which make it antiseptic, antibacterial, antiviral and antifungal, as well as pain relieving. Other monoterpenes, such as camphene, myrcene and pinene, plus sesquiterpenes (β-caryophyllene and sabinene) increase the analgesic effects.

There is a very high proportion of esters such as angelic acid, tiglic acid and methacrylic acid, which may be between 50% (Price 1993, p. 54) and 85% (Lawless 1992, p. 80). These not only add to the anti-infective effects but are also antispasmodic and relaxing. Roman camomile can be used as a relaxing massage oil in labour and will work on the digestive system to treat flatulence, heartburn, nausea and vomiting. However, due to the amount of the ketone pinocarvone (greater than the proportion of camphor in German camomile), *A. nobilis* essential oil has emmenagogic properties and *should not be used in pregnancy* until almost term. The ketones and a small amount of coumarins have anticoagulant effects, and *A. nobilis* may also stimulate both the immune system and the production of blood constituents: leucocytes to fight infection and erythrocytes to prevent anaemia. Rossi et al (1988) investigated two varieties of *A. nobilis* – 'white-headed' and 'yellow-headed' – and found the proportion of esters to be 57% in the 'white-headed' but only 33.9% in the 'yellow-headed' variety. Both oils had anti-inflammatory and sedative properties and the 'white-headed' variety was also antidiuretic. Melegari et al (1989) had similar findings.

There are small amounts of mono-alcohol in the form of bisabolol and farnesol in Roman camomile, which add to the anti-infective properties, as well as being vasoconstrictive, which makes camomile a very warming oil. Conversely, in oils produced from crops in which the proportion of sesquiterpenes such as pinocarvol is greater, there may be an antipyretic as well as a hypotensive effect. Camomile generally is a very calming and gentle oil that can safely be used on children to help them sleep.

Dangers   Camomile has emmenagogic effects so is *contraindicated in early pregnancy* and, as noted above, Roman camomile should be avoided until almost term, although Tisserand & Balacs (1995, p. 111) dispute this, suggesting that it is safe to use throughout the gestational period. Contrary to its beneficial action on the skin, a few people may develop dermatitis from prolonged use of the essential oil, as in the case of a florist who was constantly handling the plants (Van Ketel 1981), although Tisserand & Balacs (1995, p. 204) suggest there is little evidence for skin irritation. There has been a report of anaphylactic shock from camomile tea (cited by International School of Aromatherapy 1993, p. 67), and it is possible that people sensitive to camomile pollen may develop allergic rhinitis.

Blends   Either *M. chamomilla* or *A. nobilis* will blend well with benzoin, bergamot, clary sage, geranium, grapefruit, jasmine, lavender, lemon, mandarin, marjoram, neroli, orange, patchouli, rose, tangerine and ylang ylang.

Clary sage – *Salvia sclarea* (Labiatae family)

The white or blue flowers of this herb, grown in Europe and parts of America, provide the essential oil, which is extracted by steam distillation (Plate 1). The aroma is a rather heavy herbal smell, sometimes described as 'nutty'. It is important not to confuse clary sage with the more popularly known sage (Plate 2), for in aromatherapy the essential oil of sage should be used only by experienced practitioners. This is particularly significant in midwifery as there have been incidents of sage causing severe intermenstrual bleeding, menorrhagia and miscarriage.

Chemical constituents   Owing to the presence of the ester linalyl acetate, clary sage is anti-infective and acts as an uplifting nerve tonic. The alcohols linalol and sclareol are also present, adding to the antifungal, antiviral and antibacterial properties of the oil. The presence of the oxide 1,8-cineole makes clary sage a useful oil in cases of respiratory infection and congestion, for oxides are both expectorant and mucolytic; simply inhaling clary on a tissue can clear the nasal passages when one has a cold. However, the 1,8-cineole may also irritate the skin in sensitive people, so the oil should be well diluted for massage or in the bath.

The sesquiterpene caryophyllene gives clary essential oil analgesic and antispasmodic actions, so it is good for labour. Clary sage also seems to work well for premenstrual tension, dysmenorrhoea and 'after pains'. It may help with stress-related sexual problems. Unlike sage (*Salvia officinalis*), clary contains no ketones – it is the high proportion of thujone in sage which makes it a potential abortifacient and, according to Ryman (1991, p. 192) the level of thujone can be as much as 60% in the sage oil obtained from Dalmatia.

Traces of the monoterpenes myrcene, phellandrene and pinene enhance the analgesic, anti-infective and expectorant properties of the oil and act as a stimulant, but may also exacerbate any potential skin irritation, although Tisserand & Balacs (1995, p. 205) report little risk of dermal irritation in either French- or Russian-grown clary. Clary sage is certainly useful for its uplifting qualities in both labour and the postnatal period, although large doses may have the reverse effect.

Dangers   As mentioned previously, large doses of clary sage may cause headaches or drowsiness: care should be taken over the timing of administration and women should be advised not to drive immediately afterwards. Clary is known to potentiate the effects of alcohol, so should not be used shortly before or after alcohol consumption. Although clary does not contain abortifacient ketones, it is thought to be emmenagogic and therefore *should be used with caution in pregnancy* until near term.

Blends   Clary sage blends well with basil, bergamot, cedarwood, cypress, frankincense, geranium, grapefruit, jasmine, juniper berry, lavender, lime, mandarin, orange, patchouli, rose, tangerine and sandalwood.

Eucalyptus – Eucalyptus globulus (Myrtaceae family)   There are many different types of eucalyptus oil available, some such as *Eucalyptus radiata* having a camphorous aroma, others like *E. citriodora* possessing a citrussy aroma. The commonest type used is *E. globulus*, originally from Australia, although new varieties are being produced continually.

Chemical constituents   The largest proportion of any chemical in eucalyptus oil is the oxide 1,8-cineole (possibly up to 80%), making it a powerful expectorant and mucolytic but also a potential skin irritant. The alcohol globulol may be responsible for the oil's effectiveness in reducing pyrexia, while the monoterpenes camphene, fenchene, phellandrene and pinene, and the aldehyde citronellal, are antibacterial and antiviral. Consequently eucalyptus essential oil is valuable in respiratory tract infections and sinus congestion.

Tests on the antimicrobial activity of several different types of eucalyptus have shown very positive results (Gundidza et al 1993, Hajji & Fkih-Tetouani 1993, Hmamouch et al 1990, Kumar et al 1988, Low et al 1974, Penoel 1992, Zakarya et al 1993).

It is thought that there are over 250 constituents of eucalyptus oil (Ryman 1991, p. 97), including various aldehydes, terpenes and sesquiterpenic alcohols, so it is difficult to attribute the various properties to specific constituents. However, eucalyptus has also been found to be useful for urinary tract infections due to its anti-infective and diuretic effects. Adding a small amount of the oil to bathwater, deep enough to cover the suprapubic area, could be helpful for women who develop cystitis in pregnancy. Sellar (1992, p. 57) suggests that it may be of use in cases of nephritis.

Dangers   Eucalyptus is a strong essential oil, so only small doses should be used. Ingestion may lead to vomiting, central nervous system depression (Spoerke et al 1989) and even death (Leung 1980); in recounting the case of a small boy who ingested 10 ml of the oil, Patel & Wiggins (1980) quote the safe adult internal dosage as between 0.06 and 0.2 ml. Hypertensive women and epileptics (Sellar 1992, p. 57) should avoid it; use in pregnancy appears to be acceptable (Pages et al 1990), although in this latter trial the authors recognize the need for further work on the teratogenic effects.

The strong aroma of eucalyptus oil may antidote homoeopathic remedies, so the two should not be stored together, nor should anyone using homoeopathy receive simultaneous eucalyptus.

Spoerke et al's work in 1989 described 14 cases of exposure to eucalyptus essential oil. Some skin irritation occurred but subsided within 1 hour; however, it would be wise to be aware of the possible effects on the skin when using this oil. Webb & Pitt (1993) reported on 41 cases of accidental ingestion of eucalyptus by children in Australia, and although all the children recovered, this does reinforce the need to store all essential oils away from children.

Blends   Eucalyptus has an aroma that is familiar to most people and blends well with essential oils which subdue the intensity of the odour, such as benzoin, bergamot, ginger, juniper berry, lavender, lemon, melissa, tea tree and thyme.

Frankincense – *Boswellia carteri* (Burseraceae family)

With its biblical associations it is evident that frankincense has been used for many centuries as an aromatic substance in the Church as well as for perfume and, indeed, medicinally. Oleo gum resin is extracted from the bark of the tree and the essential oil is obtained through steam distillation, although an absolute is also produced for use in the perfume industry. It may be more popularly known to some readers as olibanum, a proprietary product of which is available as a decongestant. It has a camphorous aroma, as one might expect, yet is fairly light and sweet.

Chemical constituents Frankincense contains mainly monoterpenes in the form of cymene, pinene, limonene, camphene, myrcene, thujene, phellandrene and dipentene, as well as some alcohols such as farnesol, borneol, octanol, olibanol and incensol. Together these chemicals make the essential oil a strong antiseptic, which is especially good as a room purifier, and is also antibacterial, antifungal and antiviral. The antimicrobial activity of directly distilled oil has been found to be effective against some organisms such as *Staphylococcus aureus* and *Escherichia coli* but not against *Pseudomonas aeruginosa* or *Candida albicans* (Abdel Wahab et al 1987).

The monoterpenes and the alcohols are, in addition, known to be decongestant and expectorant, so the oil is very useful as an inhalation or as part of a blend for chest and back massage, for respiratory tract infections, and helps to clear the head in cases of influenza and colds.

Frankincense is reported as having an affinity with the genitourinary tract (Lawless 1992, Sellar 1992, Tisserand 1992) and can be used in the bath for women with cystitis, leucorrhoea and, in the non-pregnant woman, for dysmenorrhoea and metrorrhagia.

Frankincense is also thought to be an emmenagogue, although almost all authorities state that it is safe to use in pregnancy. Professional caution should be exercised, however, and it would be wise to use the oil only in low doses, in the absence of evidence as to its safety. In labour it can safely be used as a soothing massage oil, and postnatally may be helpful for women with depression. The presence of the alcohols means that the oil also has some vasoconstrictive effects, so theoretically making it a possible oil to use in cases of uterine haemorrhage, although this has not been demonstrated in maternity care.

Dangers Frankincense is generally considered to be a safe essential oil in all respects but, until more research is available about its emmenagogic effects, it is advisable during pregnancy to use it only in low doses.

Blends Frankincense is classed as a base note, in that its aroma is not immediately noticeable in a blend, but will linger for several hours; obviously the therapeutic effects continue to take place during this prolonged period of time. It will blend well with basil, benzoin, bergamot, black pepper, cedarwood, cinnamon, clary sage, geranium, ginger, grapefruit, jasmine, juniper berry, lavender, lemon, mandarin, melissa, myrrh, nutmeg, orange, patchouli, rosemary, rosewood, sandalwood and tangerine.

Geranium –
Pelargonium
***graveolens* or**
odorantissimum
(Geraniaceae
family)

Essential oil of geranium is distilled from the flowers of the shrub (Plate 4) to produce an oil with a rather heavy odour which may be similar to rose (*Pelargonium graveolens*) or somewhat apple-like (*P. odorantissimum*). The main producer of geranium oil is the island of Reunion, formerly known as Bourbon, and the best oil is still Bourbon geranium, although other countries are beginning to compete for production.

Chemical constituents Geranium oil has very strong anti-infective properties. The presence of alcohols such as terpenic geraniol, linalol, citronellol, borneol, myrtenol and terpineol mean that geranium is antibacterial, antifungal and antiviral, although other essential oils have been found to have a more powerful effect (Pattnaik et al 1996). Some types of geranium may exhibit antitumour activities, probably due to the citronellol, citronellyl formate, geraniol and citronellyl acetate (Fang et al 1989). The aldehyde citral and the esters geranyl acetate, linalyl acetate, citronellyl acetate, valerianic acid and acetic acid enhance these properties.

The alcohols also give the oil stimulating and uplifting qualities, although the aldehyde may have the opposite effect. In some respects geranium seems to act rather like alcohol, in exacerbating the current mood of the recipient. Too high a proportion in a blend can also lead to either hyperactivity or to a heavy soporific feeling, so care should be taken to regulate the dose. Tasev et al (1969) found that geranium, as well as rose and lavender oils, had a neuropsychic effect when tested on medical students performing a variety of tasks.

The alcohols are thought to be vasoconstrictors, which could lead to increased blood pressure, although the relaxing effects of the aldehydes, through directly working on the adrenal cortex, and of the sesquiterpenes, would appear to counteract this. In the main geranium is used as a balancer and toner, acting particularly on the reproductive and urinary tracts.

The phenol, eugenol, may induce diuresis in women with inadequate elimination processes in whom the system is congested, and geranium can be helpful in reducing oedema and toning the liver, kidneys and general circulation. The alcohols also have some effect on the liver.

A combination of terpenes such as sabinene, limonene, β-caryophyllene and phellandrene, and of eugenol (phenol), with their analgesic properties, together with the anti-inflammatory effects of geranic acid result in geranium being a useful oil for both labour and the puerperium. The oil can be blended with lavender to ease the pain of contractions during labour, although the mother should be consulted about the aroma, as a blend of these two alone may be too cloying or nauseating for some. In Lis-Balchin et al's work (1996c) 16 types of geranium oil demonstrated variable antimicrobial and antioxidant properties, but all the oils were found to be spasmolytic. It could be added to bidets and baths for perineal care postnatally as it improves the circulation, and geranium leaves have been found to be useful for sore nipples (Minchin 1994); conversely, vascular dermatitis from Bourbon geranium leaves has also been reported (International School of Aromatherapy 1993, p. 74).

Dangers   True geranium is expensive and it is possible to find cheaper brands of the oil that may have been adulterated with other essential oils such as lemongrass or cedarwood or with artificial esters (Ryman 1991, p. 106). This is important in maternity care as cedarwood not only may be a skin irritant but is also thought to be both emmenagogic and abortifacient. Consequently care should be taken when purchasing geranium to ensure its purity.

Blends   Geranium can be a very pleasant addition to many blends but is probably best used well diluted. It blends especially well with basil, bergamot, clary sage, grapefruit, jasmine, lavender, lemongrass, neroli, orange, petitgrain, rose, rosemary and sandalwood.

Ginger – *Zingiber officinale* (Zingiberaceae family)

As might be expected, ginger essential oil has a spicy, sharp, slightly woody aroma, with Jamaican ginger reputedly having the best smell. The oil is steam distilled from the dried ground root. Ginger has a very long history of medicinal use for stomach and digestive complaints in various cultures around the world.

Chemical constituents   The sesquiterpene, zingiberene, and monoterpenes, camphene, limonene and *d*-phellandrene, make ginger an effective analgesic, particularly when combined with the warming effects of the alcohols, borneol and linalol, and the oxide 1,8-cineole. Ginger also has antiseptic and anti-infective characteristics due to the aldehyde citral, the alcohols and the monoterpenes.

The carminative and digestive actions of ginger appear to arise from the presence of the 1,8-cineole and the influence on the hepatic system of the alcohols. Ginger, in either essential oil or tea form, has long been used to stimulate gastric secretions and to treat flatulence, loss of appetite, diarrhoea, and nausea and vomiting. This makes the oil valuable during pregnancy – or the mother could be advised to drink the tea or chew crystallized ginger to combat nausea. The antiemetic effects have been documented and many midwives already inform mothers about its value (Roach 1985); however the aroma can itself induce nausea in susceptible people, so care should be taken in its use.

Dangers   Ginger oil is thought to have some low-level phototoxicity. This is not significant when the oil is blended with non-phototoxic oils but may be exacerbated if mixed with phototoxic oils such as those from citrus plants. Sensitive people may develop skin irritation when the essential oil is applied in a massage blend.

Blends   Ginger will blend well with eucalyptus, frankincense, geranium, lemon, lime, orange and rosemary, with the proviso to be cautious in women with skin sensitivity.

Grapefruit – *Citrus paradisi* (Rutaceae family)

This is a lovely refreshing essence which, together with other citrus oils, lends itself especially to pregnancy and childbearing. The essence is extracted by expression of the peel of the fruit but, as the yield is less than that of orange trees, grapefruit may be slightly more expensive.

Chemical constituents   Grapefruit essence contains about 90% of the monoterpene limonene, according to Lawless (1992, p. 105), which gives it strong antiseptic and analgesic properties. The 0.0012% concentration of furocoumarins as a result of the process of extraction means that it has some phototoxic effects, although not as much as bergamot or lime (International School of Aromatherapy 1993, p. 75), and the effect can be eliminated or 'quenched' if it is blended with other non-phototoxic oils (Price 1993, p. 37), although Henson (personal communication, 1995) disputes this. It is also the furocoumarins that give the oil its calming yet refreshing effects. A 2% blend of grapefruit provides a pleasant oil for a facial or gentle abdominal massage in pregnancy.

The presence of the aldehydes citral, citronellal and neral, although in small amounts, enhance the aroma of the essence and result in the anti-inflammatory, tonic, hypotensive and depurative properties. In addition, the small quantity of geraniol, a monoterpenol (alcohol), adds to the anti-bacterial and antiviral effects of grapefruit.

Grapefruit oil has a short shelf-life of about 3 months, so should be bought in small amounts, preferably stored in the refrigerator, blended only in the quantity required and discarded after the expiry date. Antioxidant (about 0.002%) is often added to the essence to prevent premature deterioration (Price 1993, p. 89). Tisserand & Balacs (1995, p. 206) suggest that the oil should always be as fresh as possible to reduce the risk of phototoxicity.

Dangers   As with other citrus oils there is some concern regarding the phototoxicity of grapefruit, although it appears to be less severe than that of bergamot. Grapefruit should be avoided if the client is allergic to citrus fruit, otherwise it is, as far as is known, a safe and pleasant essence to use intermittently throughout pregnancy.

Blends   Grapefruit oil blends well with basil, bergamot, black pepper, camomile, clary sage, frankincense, geranium, jasmine, juniper berry, lavender, lemon, lemongrass, lime, mandarin, neroli, orange, rose, rosemary, rosewood, tangerine and ylang ylang.

**Jasmine –
*Jasminum
officinale* (Olaceae
family)**

Jasmine is probably the most expensive oil of all, making it a real luxury. It is extracted from the delicate flowers, which are picked by hand at night when their fragrance is at its most potent. The extraction process is necessarily complicated so that the flowers are not damaged; enfleurage was used originally, but jasmine oil available today is obtained by solvent extraction. The absolute is used extensively in perfumery, and indeed Ryman (1991, p. 116) suggests that today's jasmine oil is not suitable for therapeutic work partly because residual solvents will be found in the end-product. Holmes (1998) reiterates that, although the level of solvent is usually below 10 ppm, the use of jasmine absolute in aromatherapy should be restricted to dermal application in low doses. However, newer extraction methods such as the use of liquid carbon dioxide seem to have resolved the problem and most authorities continue to utilize jasmine, finding it useful in small doses of up to 2–3% (International School of Aromatherapy 1993, p. 98).

Worldwide production and availability currently exceed demand, so prices have fallen slightly since the early 1990s (Aqua Oleum 1993). Jasmine absolute is available from Egypt, India, China, Morocco, France and Algeria, with Egypt producing the most (about 70–80%) and France and Algeria the least. Concerned practitioners may, however, wish to decline from purchasing Egyptian jasmine, for, although it is likely to be the least expensive, the lower costs are achieved at the expense of local children who are paid a pittance, insufficient even to feed them for a day, to collect the flowers (Aqua Oleum 1993).

Although *Jasminum officinale* of the grandiflorum variety is the species most commonly used for the essential oils in aromatherapy, another variety, *Jasminum sambac* or Arabian jasmine, is also available.

Chemical constituents   There are well over 100 constituents in jasmine oil, which makes it difficult to synthesize, although its high price does lead to potential adulteration. It is, therefore, important to purchase the oil from a reputable supplier who can vouch for the authenticity of the batch from which you are buying.

There is a high level (about 3%) of the ketone *cis*-jasmone found in the oil, which, together with methyl anthranilate, an ester, is responsible for the sweet heady aroma. Ketones are thought to be abortifacient so jasmine *should not be used in pregnancy* until term, in the absence of evidence to the contrary.

Esters of benzyl acetate (20%, according to Holmes 1998), linalyl acetate and methyl anthranilate, and the ketones, are, however, antispasmodic so jasmine can be very useful in labour, particularly where the uterine action is inefficient, during menstruation and, following delivery, for retained placenta and 'after pains'. It has a long tradition of use in childbirth by strengthening contractions and relieving pain (the ketones and the phenol, eugenol, are analgesic), as well as being a sedative yet mood-uplifting oil.

Holmes (1998) suggests abdominal, thigh and sacral massage using jasmine in a 10–20% dilution, but in view of the general trend within clinical aromatherapy practice towards minimal dilutions, this author cannot sanction such a high dosage without further evidence of its safety. Anecdotal accounts from aromatherapists and midwives who use essential oils, as well as personal experience of the author, indicate that jasmine is *effective* in much lower doses, therefore negating the necessity of using high doses in the absence of any true evidence as to its *safety*.

It is thought to be a hormone balancer and is particularly useful for mothers with depression who could drink jasmine tea or who could be given a massage with a blend containing jasmine oil. Work by Shrivastav et al in 1988 and by Abraham et al in 1979 demonstrated the potential value of jasmine flowers in suppressing lactation. As a hormone balancer for men it may be valuable in cases of infertility, by increasing production of spermatozoa, and it is well known for its aphrodisiac qualities, in cases of frigidity, impotence and premature ejaculation (Sellar 1992, p. 81).

The oil's relaxing effect on the mind may be sedative (Davis 1988, Lawless 1992, Sellar 1992), although Tisserand (1992) states that while it is a nerve sedative it is also uplifting, and Ryman (1991) acknowledges it as a stimulant. Certainly, research by Kikuchi et al in 1989 demonstrated shortened sleeping times in mice and attributed the stimulant effects to *cis-* and *trans*-phytol. Karamat et al (1992) and Imberger et al (1993) also found jasmine to have a stimulating effect, reducing human reaction times to specified tasks and increasing concentration and attention span.

The presence of alcohols in the form of benzyl, linalol, indol, farnesol, geraniol, nerol and terpineol give jasmine its considerable anti-infective properties, including antibacterial, antifungal and antiviral effects. It is thought to be useful for respiratory tract infections, due to the presence of the ketone, jasmone.

Dangers   Jasmine has emmenagogic properties so *should not be used in pregnancy* until term. Its aroma can be overpowering for some people and overuse may result in a degree of narcosis and/or nausea: be guided by the personal preference of the mother but take care also to consider effects on birth companions and on staff. It is probably best not used in a vaporizer, except in extremely low dilutions intermittently, and because of the conflicting information regarding its sedative or stimulating effects it should be avoided at night. The cost may seem almost prohibitive to some midwives, even though the specific benefits in the care of newly delivered mothers outweigh this factor, but care must be taken that the product purchased is as pure as possible.

Blends   Jasmine is a middle note with a powerful aroma, but used in low doses will blend well with bergamot, camomile, cedarwood, clary sage, frankincense, geranium, grapefruit, lavender, lemongrass, mandarin, melissa, neroli, orange, rose, rosewood, sandalwood, tangerine and ylang ylang.

Juniper berry –
Juniperus
communis
(Cupressaceae family)

Juniper berry essential oil, produced from *Juniperus communis*, must not be confused with oil from other species of juniper, such as *J. virginiana* from which Virginian cedarwood oil is obtained, or *J. sabina* which produces savin oil. Savin oil may have some adverse effects in pregnancy, as shown by preliminary work in mice by Pages et al (1989), although later work (1996) by the same researchers found anti-implantation effects to be responsible for its abortifacient action but no impaired fertility or increased fetal malformations. The oils from both *J. virginiana* and *J. sabina* contain a different balance of chemicals that may be detrimental to a client for whom oil from *J. communis* is appropriate.

The essential oil is extracted from the berries and other parts of the bush by steam distillation, producing a refreshing aroma with a hint of woodiness. Another oil is also produced from *J. communis*: juniper needle oil. This has a high sabinene content, whereas juniper berry is rich in α-pinene.

Chemical constituents   The essential oil is rich in monoterpenes (camphene, pinene, myrcene, phellandrene and limonene) and in sesquiterpenes (cadinene, sabinene, cymene and terpinene). Together these chemicals result in juniper berry being useful as a disinfectant and antiseptic. The sesquiterpenes give it anti-inflammatory and antispasmodic properties, although Lis–Balchin et al's work (1996b) could not substantiate this claim, and help in lowering the blood pressure.

The main functions of juniper berry seem to be diuretic, probably due to an increase in the glomerular filtration rate, enabling more sodium and potassium to be excreted (Tisserand 1992, p. 242). This means that it could be very useful in cases of severe ankle oedema in the postnatal period when the autolytic processes of involution, working faster than renal excretion, result in exacerbation of any pre-existing oedema. However, juniper berry is also an emmenagogue and should therefore *not* be used for oedematous ankles during pregnancy, except *perhaps* near term (see below).

Juniper berry also contains alcohols such as borneol and terpineol, which add to the antibacterial and antiviral properties, as well as acting on the hepatic system which may help with detoxification of the liver, and it has apparently been used in cases of cirrhosis. Urinary tract infection in the puerperium may respond well to juniper berry in combination with other oils. Stassi (1996) investigated four different types of juniper berry and found them to be active against a range of organisms.

Dangers   Juniper berry is known to be an emmenagogue and should perhaps be used with caution in pregnancy, although Tisserand & Balacs (1995, p. 110) argue that this is not a reason for not using it. They cite several studies that refer to juniper generically and do not identify *J. communis* specifically. They acknowledge that juniper berries are known to be abortifacient but this does not seem to apply to the essential oil. A comprehensive discussion of their reasons for disputing the contraindication of juniper berries in pregnancy is given in their *Essential Oil Safety* guide (1995, p. 142), but it is the belief of this author that, until more definite evidence is available, those caring for pregnant women should be extremely circumspect about the use of juniper berries during pregnancy, and ensure that they are using only *J. communis*.

The effects on the renal tract have not been fully investigated, and juniper berry should not be used on women who have a history of renal disease (International School of Aromatherapy 1993, p. 65), including gestational hypertension. Overuse in women with no history of kidney disease *may* precipitate renal complications, although, again, Tisserand & Balacs (1995, p. 142) suggest that as long as the oil is truly good quality *J. communis*, it is not contraindicated in either pregnancy or kidney disease. They claim that there are no contraindications, no risk of oral, dermal or phototoxicity, but that the oil used should be fresh (Tisserand & Balacs 1995, p. 206).

Prolonged use may result in allergy to the skin and respiratory tract, although the case reported by Rothe et al in 1973 occurred after 25 years of occupational contact with products containing *J. communis*. Neat application of juniper berry oil may have approximately 2% incidence of irritation (International School of Aromatherapy 1993, p. 65).

Blends   Juniper berry will blend well with benzoin, bergamot, cedarwood, clary sage, cypress, eucalyptus, frankincense, geranium, grapefruit, lemon, lime, melissa, orange, rosemary, sandalwood and thyme.

Lavender –
Lavandula
angustifolia
(Labiatae family)

Lavender is probably the most versatile essential oil used in aromatherapy and is produced by steam distillation from the flowers, and occasionally the stalks. The word 'lavender' originates from the Latin 'to wash', and the plant has a long worldwide tradition of medicinal usage as a cleanser. The quality of lavender varies according to the place in which it is grown, with some of the best coming from Grasse in France, the Alps, Norfolk in England and the former Yugoslavia.

There are, however, several types of lavender oil available and this is particularly important in maternity care. *Lavandula angustifolia*, sometimes known as *L. officinalis*, is the most odorous and the most commonly used therapeutic oil.

Practitioners should always ask for the oil by its Latin name to avoid being offered one of the other types of lavender such as *L. stoechas, L. vera, L. dentata* (this latter is rich in 1,8-cineole as shown by Gamez et al's work in 1990) or even *L. spica* or *latifolia*, more usually called spike lavender. *L. intermedia, hortensis* and *burnatii* are terms that refer to essential oil of lavandin, obtained from a hybrid cross between *L. angustifolia* and *L. latifolia*. Lavandin oil is much cheaper to produce than lavender and is sometimes substituted for the latter, but the chemical constituents differ considerably. Other oils are occasionally mistaken for lavender: the cotton lavender is actually *Santolina chamaecyparissus*, belonging to an entirely different botanical family and having no use in aromatherapy because of its potential toxicity, including dangers from oral use during pregnancy, fever or in people with epilepsy.

A trial by Buckle (1993) investigated the different effects of *L. officinalis* and *L. burnatii* on patients after cardiac surgery. She found that respiratory effects were similar but that *L. burnatii* appeared to be more effective in alleviating anxiety. It was noted that lavandin oil is rarely used (although trials into the antimycobacterial activity of lavandin have also been carried out by Gabbrielli et al (1988)). While there were some flaws in the methodology of Buckle's trial, it was one of the first randomized double-blind controlled investigations in therapeutic aromatherapy and serves to demonstrate the importance of selecting essential oils by their Latin name rather than their common name.

Chemical constituents   *L. angustifolia* contains alcohols such as linalol, borneol, geraniol and lavandulol, which together with some phenols makes it a strong anti-infective agent. Lavender is thought to be antibacterial, antifungal, antiviral and antimicrobial, and could be effective in reducing wound infection in mothers following Caesarean section or episiotomy. Piccaglia et al (1993) found lavender to be particularly effective against *Clostridium sporogenes* and *Staphylococcus aureus*. Perruci et al (1996) demonstrated lavender's effectiveness in killing parasites. Dale & Cornwell's (1994) trial involving 635 women did not in fact demonstrate significant anti-infective effects of lavender oil used postepisiotomy, nor did there appear to be more rapid wound healing, another property attributed to lavender oil. However, the mothers did report a decrease in discomfort, and lavender is noted to be an effective analgesic, notably for headaches, due to its phenol and terpene (limonene, pinene and caryophyllene, a sesquiterpene) content. Consequently it can be useful in labour for easing contraction pain, and also acts as an antispasmodic due to the presence of esters such as geranyl acetate, lavandulyl acetate and linalyl acetate. Experience has shown that lavender oil massaged into the abdomen and back during labour seems to enhance and coordinate uterine action and can be effective where the placenta is slow to separate in the third stage of labour. In addition the phenols and esters produce a feeling of relaxation and sedation, as shown in work by Buchbauer et al (1991, 1993), Guillemain et al (1989), Karamat et al (1992) and Sugano & Sato (1991). Lavender has also been shown to have anticonvulsant properties when inhaled (Yamada et al 1994).

Lavender oil is hypotensive due to the alcohols and sesquiterpenes, and can be valuable in late pregnancy and in labour where a mother has raised blood pressure. However, it should be used with caution for women with epidural anaesthesia *in situ* as it may compound the possible hypotensive effects of bupivacaine.

Lavender oil contains a small amount of the ketone camphor, which can be emmenagogic, as well as some 1,8-cineole, an oxide, so, contrary to popular belief, lavender is *should be used with caution in early pregnancy*, although some texts suggest that it may be used in small doses for conditions such as leucorrhoea. Percutaneous absorption of the oil into the blood has been demonstrated within 10 minutes of administration (Jager et al 1992), although after 90 minutes most of the lavender had been eliminated from the blood of subjects in the trial. This may or may not have implications for its use in early pregnancy, although many authorities see no reason to place restrictions on it. The expectorant action of the oxide content does, however, make lavender a good addition to an inhalation for respiratory tract congestion and infection.

Dangers   As noted above, lavender oil should be administered with caution, in low doses, intermittently in early pregnancy. Care should be taken that the oil used is *L. angustifolia* – be guided by price. Some dermal irritation has been reported (Brandao 1986), although dermal toxicity of spike lavender (*L. spica*) is more than twice that of *L. angustifolia* (International School of Aromatherapy 1993, p. 74), again emphasizing the need to be sure of the product being purchased. This advice is given by implication by Tisserand & Balacs (1995, p. 231), who state that oral, rectal and vaginal administration of lavandin, *L. stoechas* and spike lavender is contraindicated.

The hypotensive action should be carefully monitored, and this, coupled with the sedating effects, may make some people feel drowsy after use. Certainly the hypotensive action precludes the use of lavender in women prone to postural hypotension or possibly in those receiving epidural anaesthesia.

Blends   Lavender has a very distinctive aroma, liked by most people, but some may prefer it to be subdued by blending with other oils. Lavender mixes well with basil, benzoin, bergamot, camomile, cedarwood, cinnamon, clary sage, cypress, eucalyptus, frankincense, geranium, grapefruit, jasmine, lemon, lemongrass, lime, mandarin, marjoram, melissa, neroli, nutmeg, orange, patchouli, petitgrain, rose, rosemary, rosewood, sandalwood, tangerine, tea tree, thyme and ylang ylang.

Lemon – *Citrus limon* Burman (Rutaceae family)   As might be expected, lemon essential oil has a lovely fresh citrussy aroma and is obtained by expression from the rind of the fruit. Ryman (1991, p. 129) states that production of lemon essence is second only to orange and that in 1987 2000–2500 tonnes of the oil were produced worldwide. This was superseded in 1991 when over 10 000 tonnes were produced

(Aqua Oleum 1993). Much of the therapeutic value of the oil can be obtained by ingesting the fruit or in part from drinking the juice, especially for its vitamin C content, but the essential oil has been used for many centuries as an antiseptic.

Chemical constituents   The principal constituent of lemon oil is limonene, a monoterpene, in quantities up to 70% (Lawless 1992, p. 119) or even 90%, (Wattenberg & Coccia 1991), together with other monoterpenes myrcene, phellandrene and pinene, and some sesquiterpenes in the form of sabinene, cadinene, terpinene and β-bisabolene. The terpenes, in combination with alcohols (geraniol, linalol, nonalol, octanol) and the aldehyde, citral, mean that lemon is anti-infective, antiseptic, antifungal, antibacterial and antiviral. Research by Subba et al in 1967 showed that lemon was not as effective an oil against a range of microorganisms as orange oil, although later work by Misra et al (1988) demonstrated lemon's antifungal activity, with citral being found to be the most effective component. Lemon is also considered to be an immunostimulant, increasing the production of leucocytes, and may possibly improve erythrocyte vitality, thereby preventing anaemia. Work by Wattenberg & Coccia (1991) on mice indicates a potential anticarcinogenic property of lemon, orange and *d*-limonene.

The alcohols have a vasoconstrictive action and lemon has been used as a haemostatic agent in cases of haemorrhage. However, it is also thought to be a tonic to the circulatory system and may be effective in reducing hypertension, probably due to the alcohols, in conjunction with the coumarins and aldehydes. In addition, the coumarins seem to have an anticoagulant action, while the alcohols may act on the hepatic system.

Lemon does appear to work in almost a homoeopathic manner, for despite its acidic nature it can be helpful in reducing hyperacidity of the gastrointestinal tract. It is certainly known to be an effective laxative oil.

The fresh aroma is virtually universally pleasing and may act directly on the brain through the olfactory tract as an antidepressant and an uplift to the emotions, as demonstrated by Knasko's (1992) work.

Dangers   Much has been written about the possible phototoxic effects of lemon essence, as well as other citrus essences, thought in this case to be due to the presence of bergapten and oxypeucedanin (Naganuma et al 1985) although Tisserand & Balacs (1995, p. 87) state that expressed lemon oil contains only 0.15–0.25% bergapten compared with 0.3–0.4% in bergamot oil. Certainly lemon oil should not be used neat on the skin; dermatitis is possible in sensitive people, and low doses of about 1–2% are recommended. Audicana & Bernaola (1994) report on the potentially serious skin complaints which may arise as a result of frequent contact with lemons and other citrus fruits; they attributed the effects to the *d*-limonene and suggest patch testing may be appropriate.

Oxidization can occur in lemon oil left exposed to oxygen or light, so it is best to buy small quantities of a good quality oil, ensuring that its shelf-life is still valid at the time of purchase.

Blends   The fresh aroma of lemon essence will counteract some of the very heavy base aromas, and will blend well with benzoin, bergamot, black pepper, camomile, cedarwood, cypress, eucalyptus, frankincense, geranium, ginger, grapefruit, jasmine, juniper berry, lavender, mandarin, neroli, nutmeg, orange, patchouli, petitgrain, rose, sandalwood, tangerine, tea tree, thyme and ylang ylang.

Lemongrass – *Cymbopogon citratus* (Gramineae family)   The oil is steam distilled from the grass, which is grown in the tropics, and much of the production is used by the food and perfumery industries. It is occasionally called Indian melissa or Indian verbena, but this must not be confused with *Melissa officinalis* or *Lippia citriodora*, respectively.

Chemical constituents   Lemongrass oil contains up to 85% of the aldehyde citral, which is responsible for a strong antifungal and bactericidal action (Agarwal et al 1980, Ogunlana et al 1987, Onawunmi, 1988, 1989, Onawunmi & Ogunlana 1986, Onawunmi et al 1984), although this is reduced by oxidization of the oil as a result of exposure to light, heat and oxygen (Orafidiya 1993). Analgesia owing to the monoterpenes, limonene and myrcene, has been demonstrated by Lorenzetti et al (1991), while Seth et al (1976) found the oil not only to relieve pain but also to be antipyretic and a central nervous system depressant. It is quoted as helping to eliminate lactic acid following exercise (Sellar 1992, p. 92), although there is no scientific evidence to support this claim, but it could be of use during labour and the postnatal period as a means of refreshing and uplifting the mother, thereby facilitating her to draw on her own reserves of energy. It is also galactogogic, so may help in establishing lactation, although Tisserand & Balacs (1995, p. 230) advise caution if the oil is administered orally to breastfeeding women. Indeed, they advise that the oral route of administration of the essential oil should also be with caution in people with glaucoma (1995, p. 146). These precautions do not, however, appear to relate to the use of whole lemongrass in cooking.

Citral and the alcohol geraniol have been found to reduce serum cholesterol levels (Elson et al 1989) and lemongrass seems to have a carminative action, aiding digestion, stimulating appetite, relieving heartburn and easing flatulence. Other alcohols present include citronellol, farnesol, furfurol, geraniol, isopulegol, linalol, nerol and terpineol. Some anticarcinogenic qualities have been attributed to lemongrass oil, possibly because of the geraniol and *d*-limonene content (Zheng et al 1993).

Emotionally, the clean refreshing aroma of the oil seems to act in lifting the spirits and reviving energy. Lemongrass is an effective deodorant and insect repellant, and could be vaporized intermittently into the maternity department as an air freshener.

Dangers Oxidization can occur fairly rapidly because of the high proportion of citral which changes to an acid and therefore affects the chemical profile of the oil, rendering it unsuitable for therapeutic work; Orafidiya (1993) found that autoxidation rendered the lemongrass oil inactive against *E. coli* and *S. aureus.* There is some risk of dermal irritation as a result of the citral content so the oil should be used only in low dilutions.

Lemongrass oil should be avoided in children under the age of 2 years. As a related issue Tisserand & Balacs (1995, p. 230) advise caution in women with endometriosis probably as endometriosis could be exacerbated by oestrogenic essential oils, especially when given orally.

Blends Lemongrass blends well with basil, cedarwood, eucalyptus, geranium, jasmine, juniper berry, lavender, neroli, patchouli, rosemary and tea tree.

Lime – *Citrus aurantifolia* (Rutaceae family) Lime is a much under-rated essential oil, and is valuable in maternity care as a member of the citrus group, with its fresh, sweet aroma, similar to bergamot. It should not be confused with lime blossom, sometimes called linden blossom (*Tilia europaea* or *cordata*), which is completely different. Unlike most citrus fruits, expression is not the principal method of extraction, although it may be used to produce oil for the perfumery industry; the essential oil for aromatherapy is normally obtained from the whole fruit by steam distillation, as the expressed product is phototoxic.

Chemical constituents As might be expected, lime, in common with other citrus oils, contains limonene (between 42 and 64% according to Tisserand & Balacs (1995, p. 147)) and other monoterpenes such as camphene and pinene as well as sequiterpenes in the form of sabinene and terpinoline. These give the oil strong antiseptic and anti-infective properties, and are also responsible for the relaxing yet uplifting quality so easily evoked by simply inhaling the aroma.

The alcohols linalol and terpineol and the aldehyde citral also assist in the antibacterial, antiviral, antifungal and antiseptic actions of lime oil. In addition alcohols are thought to balance the immune system and act on the liver, possibly being useful in treating alcoholism (Sellar 1992, p. 95). The terpenes, alcohols and aldehydes all contribute towards the relaxing effect of lime, while aldehydes and alcohols can help in reducing pyrexia.

Esters such as linalyl acetate, together with the sesquiterpenes, make lime oil anti-inflammatory and antispasmodic, so it is a good all-round choice for labour.

Lime is also used as an appetite regulator and could be beneficial for women with loss of appetite or with pica, as well as those suffering ptyalism. Lime, with or without ginger oil, can often be useful in easing pregnancy sickness; alternatively women could be advised to try lime juice cordial.

Lime oil is considered safe to use throughout pregnancy (International School of Aromatherapy 1993, p. 146) and could be blended with other citrus essences or alternated with them according to the woman's preference.

Dangers   As with all citrus oils there is a risk of photosensitivity, although judicious use should reduce the potential dangers. High doses may irritate the skin in susceptible women.

Blends   Lime oil blends well with all the other citrus essences such as bergamot, lemon, mandarin, orange, tangerine and petitgrain. It also complements citronella, clary sage, lavender, lemongrass, neroli, nutmeg, rose, rosemary and ylang ylang.

Mandarin – *Citrus nobilis* (Rutaceae family)

Mandarin has a lovely fresh citrus aroma reminiscent of the actual fruit and is obtained by cold expression from the outer peel. Mandarin is one of the most versatile and gentlest of essential oils and, as far as is known, is suitable for use on almost anyone receiving aromatherapy but particularly expectant mothers and children.

Chemical constituents   Mandarin essence has a bluish tinge owing to the presence of methyl anthranilate, an ester which makes it a good antiseptic. It has an affinity with the gastrointestinal tract, being carminative, digestive and laxative as a result of the esters. The aldehydes citral and citronellal and the alcohol geraniol provide the anti-infective properties of the essence. In addition geraniol assists diuresis while the esters are antispasmodic. A small amount of the monoterpene limonene gives mandarin essence analgesic properties but is also responsible for the potential to cause skin irritation. Conversely it can be useful in reducing the tendency to striae gravidarum and scarring. Like all citrus essences, mandarin is thought to be slightly phototoxic but this has not been shown to be significant.

Mandarin's refreshing aroma is almost universally acceptable and, as it is safe and versatile, it can be used on virtually all clients except those allergic to citrus fruit. The terpenes act as a stimulant and mild antidepressant, the latter characteristic being enhanced by the phenols.

Dangers   As mentioned above, mandarin may be phototoxic if used undiluted and could cause some skin irritation in sensitive people, but is otherwise one of the safest essences to use in aromatherapy. Care should, however, be taken, as with all essential oils, not to use it continuously throughout pregnancy; in labour its use should be intermittent and midwives should consider discontinuing it if the mother is having an emotionally unsatisfying labour, in an attempt to prevent long-term olfactory association of mandarin with an unpleasant situation.

Blends   Mandarin blends well with many essential oils including basil, bergamot, black pepper, camomile, grapefruit, lavender, lemon, lemongrass, lime, marjoram, neroli, nutmeg, petitgrain, rose, rosemary, sandalwood, tea tree and ylang ylang.

Marjoram – *Origanum marjorana* (Labiatae family)

This oil, with its warm, spicy and somewhat medicinal aroma, is produced by distillation from the flowers and leaves of the plant (Plate 5). It has a long tradition of use as a medicine, especially for stomach upsets.

Chemical constituents   The alcohols, borneol, linalol, pinocarvol and α-terpineol, mean that marjoram is a good anti-infective agent, being antibacterial, antifungal and antiviral, as well as an immune system balancer (Deans & Svoboda 1990). They also act directly on the hepatic system, helping to stimulate and aid liver and biliary function, and can be helpful in alleviating constipation and abdominal colic. The monoterpene pinene and the sesquiterpenes sabinene and β-caryophyllene assist in relieving pain, especially muscular discomfort following exercise, and headache. Camphor, a ketone, is a valuable expectorant, so is useful for colds, influenza and bronchitis, but is also an emmenagogue so marjoram *should be avoided in pregnancy*, except in very small doses towards term.

Aldehydes, in the form of citral and geranyl acetate, add to the anti-infective qualities of the oil, and also lower the blood pressure; this is enhanced by the large number of alcohols. In addition, aldehydes help to lower temperature, and are relaxing, but may be responsible for skin irritation.

Phenolic glycosides, arbutin and hydroquinone, have been found in Egyptian marjoram oil, and the latter component showed some cytotoxic activity against cultured rat cells (Assaf et al 1987).

Dangers   Marjoram should be *avoided in early pregnancy* as insufficient information is known about its emmenagogic properties. The relaxing effects may be sufficient to cause drowsiness, so care should be taken when using marjoram that the client is not about to drive a vehicle. Consideration may also need to be given to staff exposed to the vapours as the relaxing effects could potentially impair professional judgement.

When purchasing the oil it is important not to confuse *Origanum majorana* (commonly called sweet marjoram) with Spanish marjoram (*Thymus mastichina*), which has a much higher 1,8-cineole content, sometimes up to 75%.

Blends   Marjoram has a warm camphorous aroma which blends well with basil, bergamot, camomile, cedarwood, clary sage, cypress, lavender, lemon, mandarin, melissa, nutmeg, orange, peppermint, rosewood and sandalwood.

Neroli – *Citrus aurantium* or *bigaradia* (Rutaceae family)

This is one of the most expensive and luxurious essential oils, derived from the delicate petals of the bitter orange tree by a process of solvent extraction or occasionally steam distillation from the freshly picked flowers – a tonne of flowers is needed to produce just one kilogram of oil, hence the price.

Chemical constituents   Neroli contains a high proportion of alcohols (linalol, nerol, nerolidol, farnesol, indol, terpineol and geraniol), as well as esters such as linalyl acetate, methyl anthranilate, geranyl acetate, benzyl acetate and neryl acetate. There is a small amount of the ketone, jasmone, and some monoterpenes in the form of limonene, α- and β-pinene, and camphene.

The main value of neroli appears to be reduction of stress, a result of the relaxing properties of the esters, aldehydes and ketones, and the hypotensor effects of the alcohols and aldehydes. Stevenson's (1992) controlled trial with patients in intensive care demonstrated that relaxation and reduction in anxiety could be obtained from a 10-minute foot massage using neroli.

Jager et al (1992) also demonstrated reduced motility, i.e. sedation, in mice as did Buchbauer et al (1993). This oil could certainly be used in pregnancy in small doses, and particularly in labour to alleviate tension and stress. Ryman (1991, p. 155) recommends its use for premenstrual tension, and this could equally apply to postnatal 'blues' and depression. The esters are responsible for neroli being antispasmodic, which may be further justification for its use during labour, involution and subsequent menstruation.

Neroli has been quoted as being aphrodisiac (Lawless 1992, p. 144), possibly as a result of the relaxation obtained, and this would make it a suitable oil for women to use after the puerperium when their libido may not have returned to normal.

For insomnia during late pregnancy or the puerperium neroli is a special oil to add to a blend, although it can have a rather hypnotic effect on some people.

The toning effect on the circulatory system is possibly due to the high level of alcohols, and neroli seems to assist in promoting healthy skin. During late pregnancy abdominal massage with neroli oil *may* prevent striae gravidarum although it is probable that women prone to striae will be unable to prevent them totally, and can promote wound healing and cell regeneration in the postnatal period.

Dangers   Neroli is thought to be safe to use in pregnancy but it is advisable to blend it in low dilutions owing to the presence of a small amount of jasmone. The relaxation achieved can be soporific and hypnotic, so women should not drive immediately after receiving it.

Blends   Neroli is a base note with an aroma that takes a while to warm up and which lingers longer than many other orangey aromas. It blends well with basil, bergamot, camomile, cedarwood, citronella, geranium, jasmine, lemon, lemongrass, lime, mandarin, melissa, orange, patchouli, petitgrain, rose, sandalwood, tangerine and ylang ylang.

Nutmeg – *Myristica fragrans* (Myristicaceae family)

Essential oil of nutmeg is obtained from the seed kernels by steam distillation and has a warm spicy, rather sharp, aroma. The UK is quoted (Ryman 1991, p. 158) as being the second largest consumer of nutmeg oil in the world. The essential oil should be very pale yellow with a thin consistency; if it has turned dark brown, thick and has a more unpleasant aroma, it should not be used for therapeutic work.

Chemical constituents   Nutmeg oil contains between 1 and 14% of the phenol myristicine, depending on its source. This can not only cause severe skin irritation but is also narcotic, hallucinogenic and toxic, and for this reason the oil should certainly *never be used in pregnancy* – the fact that it is also an emmenagogue is less significant than the overall toxicity of the oil. Tisserand & Balacs (1995, p. 107) dispute this and suggest that administration via massage is acceptable, there being insufficient proof regarding the need to avoid it during pregnancy. It is, however, this very lack of evidence that should govern its use – or lack of use – in maternity care.

Other phenols present include safrole (which is potentially carcinogenic, although work by Bannerjee et al (1994) indicate that nutmeg may have some anticarcinogenic activity) and eugenol, so that nutmeg is a powerful anti-infective oil. Bennett et al's work (1988) demonstrated that the eugenol reduces muscle tone in the gastrointestinal tract and myometrium, and inhibits prostaglandin synthesis. It also appears to have anti-inflammatory effects and has been used for many years as an effective treatment for diarrhoea. Later investigations by Janssens et al (1990) showed that eugenol and isoeugenol are effective in inhibiting platelet aggegration, but they recommended that, to prevent the side-effects of nutmeg oil, synthetic preparations of the active ingredients should be used in preference.

The carminative, laxative phenols generally mean that nutmeg is good for digestive complaints, including both diarrhoea and constipation.

Various alcohols (about 4–8% according to Lawless (1992, p. 139)) such as geraniol, borneol, linalol, cymol, sapol, globulol and terpineol add to the antibacterial, antiviral and antifungal properties, and act as an immune system balancer. Alcohols are also vasoconstrictive and nutmeg is known to be a cardiac stimulant, so should never be used in high doses.

Up to 88% of the oil is comprised of the monoterpenes camphene, dipentene, pinene, limonene and phellandrene, and the sesquiterpenes, α-terpenene and sabinene, which give nutmeg strong analgesic properties that seem especially effective for uterine pain in labour or for dysmenorrhoea; indeed, nutmeg has a tradition in some cultures of being used for childbearing women. This author has had experience of using nutmeg to induce labour (with obstetric consultant permission only) or accelerate uterine action, often only needing to use one drop. However, non-midwifery-qualified aromatherapists are reminded of their parameters of accountable practice and should *not* resort to attempting to induce labour.

Tisserand & Balacs (1995, p. 153) cite research which demonstrates that nutmeg's main constituent, myristicin, inhibits monoamine oxidase, although this is less significant in the whole essential oil. However, mono-amine oxidase inhibitors should not be given in conjunction with pethidine (Reynolds 1993), so if nutmeg oil is used during labour the midwife should make the mother aware that she will not be able to resort to pethidine simultaneously. It is also good for other muscular aches and pains, notably rheumatic and dental pain. The presence of the oxide 1,8-cineole means that the oil is expectorant and mucolytic.

As an anti-stress remedy nutmeg has been used for many years, and recently an American company has patented the oil following investigations into its use in reducing blood pressure (Aqua Oleum 1993).

Dangers   The myristicin content of nutmeg oil makes it potentially lethal in aromatherapy. It is included here because, in experienced hands, small doses of the oil can be of use during labour, except in women also receiving pethidine. Many texts on aromatherapy seem to contradict one another as to the safety of nutmeg oil, but with the current level of knowledge it is advised that it should *not be used in pregnancy* and the maximum dilution recommended is 2% in fit healthy adults.

Tests on animals have shown central nervous system paralysis and fatty degeneration of the liver (Balacs 1993); intoxication in humans can lead to nausea and vomiting, tachycardia, visual impairment, stupor, epileptiform fits and hallucinations (International School of Aromatherapy 1993, p. 79). Farrell (1994) cites the report of a 25-year-old man with acute psychosis as a result of chronic nutmeg abuse. The danger of ingesting the oil should be remembered, too, when storing it, particularly when in the home, for overdose in a child could be fatal. It is interesting to note that mice given large amounts of Coca-Cola, which also contains myristicin, developed hepatic problems associated with carcinogenicity, although the researchers did point out that there is no direct evidence of the carcinogenic tendency of myristicin-containing essential oils (Balacs 1993).

Blends   Nutmeg can be used in small doses by experienced aromatherapists who also fully understand the physiology of labour, and blends well with black pepper, cinnamon, clary sage, cypress, frankincense, geranium, lemon, lime, mandarin, melissa, orange, patchouli, petitgrain, rosemary and tea tree.

**Orange, sweet –
Citrus sinensis
(Rutaceae family)**   Sweet orange is one of the safest and most versatile of all the essences and can be used during pregnancy and for children. It is obtained from the rind by cold expression or steam distillation, but, because it can oxidize quickly, antioxidants are usually added.

A similar oil is obtained from the bitter orange peel (*Citrus aurantium*) but the larger amount of coumarins increases the potential phototoxic effects of the bitter orange essence.

Chemical constituents   As with other citrus essences, sweet orange contains over 90% of monoterpenes, mainly limonene, with some camphene, myrcene and the sesquiterpene sabinene. These assist in the antiseptic and antibacterial qualities of sweet orange but also contribute towards the possible skin irritation that may occur in some people when sweet orange is used in high doses.

Aldehydes in the form of citral, together with the esters methyl anthranilate and neryl acetate, some coumarins and alcohols (fenchol, terpineol, linalol and nerol) make orange a relaxing essence and a mood uplifter, suitable for administration to women with hypertension, insomnia, anxiety, stress and depression. It is possible that it could be of value for hypercholesterolaemia.

Sweet orange is one of the most valuable essences to use for digestive complaints including nausea and vomiting, especially of biliary aetiology, constipation, diarrhoea, lack of appetite and possibly weight loss through its effect on fats. It can be used for babies with colic too.

The vitamin C content is obviously helpful for colds and influenza, although it would be better to eat whole oranges or drink the fresh juice. However, the essence may be effective in reducing pyrexia, probably by inducing sweating.

The essence can have a beneficial action on the skin and may help to prevent or reduce the severity of striae gravidarum, dry skin and dermatitis.

The analgesic effects of the monoterpenes indicate orange essence's value in labour. It is thought to reduce oedema, so could be good to use in late pregnancy and in the early puerperium for swollen ankles and feet (it is certainly safer than some other oils used to reduce oedema), and could be used during the premenstrual phase or the menopause.

Dangers   Sweet orange is extremely versatile and, as far as is known, safe to use in almost anyone. However, it should not be used in people who are allergic to citrus fruit. Neither should its versatility lead to prolonged use, as no oil should be used continuously for more than 3 weeks.

Care should be taken to purchase *Citrus sinensis* and to ensure it is as organic as possible, for many crops of oranges are sprayed with chemicals to improve their colour, or with wax to help retain moisture. Only small quantities of the essence should be purchased as it will deteriorate quickly and must be stored in a cool dark place with the lid of the bottle firmly in place. When blending, only the amount required should be mixed and any left over discarded.

There is a risk of skin irritation in some women with sensitive skins, and phototoxicity may be a problem if the woman goes into bright sunlight immediately after administration, although it is likely that the effects last no longer than 2 hours.

Blends   The refreshing, sweet and familiar aroma of oranges is pleasing to almost everyone. However, care should be taken as to how it is used, especially during labour, for if labour and delivery are difficult or unsatisfying for the mother, she may reject oranges for life because of olfactory memory.

Sweet orange blends well with basil, benzoin, bergamot, camomile, cinnamon, clary sage, cypress, frankincense, geranium, ginger, grapefruit, jasmine, juniper berry, lavender, lemon, lemongrass, lime, mandarin, marjoram, neroli, nutmeg, patchouli, petitgrain, rose, rosemary, rosewood, sandalwood, tangerine, tea tree and ylang ylang.

Patchouli – *Pogostemon patchouli* (Labiatae family)

Patchouli oil is extracted from the leaves by steam distillation, and the heavy sweet aroma improves with age, lingering for a long time once used (hence it is a base note, often used in perfumery as a fixative). It may be a yellowish brown in colour or a deep reddish brown due to iron deposits oxidized from the metal containers in which it is stored when distilled in its country of origin (Seychelles, Indonesia, China and India). Patchouli has a long tradition of use in Chinese and Indian medicine and some readers may recall the 'Swinging Sixties' when it was often burned as incense with sandalwood and jasmine.

Chemical constituents   About 40% of the oil is comprised of the alcohol patchoulol; Yang et al (1996) found 41% of patchoulol in Chinese patchouli compared with 20–23% in Indian and Indonesian patchouli oils. There are around 18% esters and sesquiterpenes in the form of patchoulene, caryophyllene and cadinene, aldehydes such as benzoic and cinnamic aldehyde, with the phenol eugenol, make up the bulk of the remaining constituents. There is also a small amount of the ketone carvone present in the oil and up to 40% patchouli camphor in the dried leaves (Ryman 1991, p. 171). Davis (1988, p. 259) notes that patchoulene has a similar chemical structure to azulene, produced from camomile during the extraction process, which may account for the comparable anti-inflammatory properties of patchouli.

The oil can be sedative in action when used in low doses but may have the reverse effect when the concentration is too high. Some authorities suggest it has aphrodisiac properties and can help in increasing libido, while others question this as the aroma can be unpleasant for some people, especially in larger doses. It is often quoted as being an antidepressant.

Patchouli oil appears to be effective for use on the skin, easing allergies and eczema, and helping with wound healing when the skin is cracked, possibly by encouraging tissue regeneration and scar formation. The anti-infective properties are particularly useful for fungal infections of the skin such as athlete's foot, and for scalp conditions such as dandruff. It may also be of help for haemorrhoids.

Several authorities believe that patchouli oil can be effective in treating obesity by curbing appetite, acting as a diuretic and preventing fluid retention and cellulite. It has been used for both diarrhoea by toning the gastrointestinal tract and for constipation by stimulating a sluggish colon (Tisserand 1992, p. 264).

Dangers   Ryman comments (1991, p. 171) that no research has been undertaken to evaluate the effects of the iron that leaches from the metal containers used for storage, or of the second distillation often carried out by perfumers in an attempt to alter the colour, on the therapeutic actions of the final oil. Occasionally the oil may be adulterated with others such as cedar or cubebs, or with synthetic caryophyllene.

Care should be taken with dosage to ensure the correct balance and to avoid stimulating the central nervous system when sedation is the required effect.

No authorities appear to have questioned the use of patchouli specifically during pregnancy and it is not considered to be an emmenagogue, but it would be wise to be cognisant of the various effects and to use the oil sparingly.

Blends   The aroma of patchouli may be too heavy for some women and the therapist should be guided by the preference of the individual. The oil blends well with bergamot, black pepper, clary sage, frankincense, geranium, ginger, lavender, lemongrass, neroli, orange, rose, rosewood and sandalwood.

Petitgrain – *Citrus bigaradia* (Rutaceae family)

Petitgrain essential oil is extracted by steam distillation from the leaves and twigs of the bitter orange tree from which neroli is also derived, and contemporary supplies come from Paraguay, although small quantities of a better quality oil still come from France. The essential oil is used extensively in both the perfumery and the food industries, but not a great deal in aromatherapy. However, it does have some therapeutic values and, as far as is known, is safe to use in pregnancy.

Chemical constituents   The oil contains up to 80% esters such as linalyl acetate, geranyl acetate, neryl acetate and terpenyl acetate, but oxidization can cause these to convert to acids so care must be taken to store the oil appropriately. The esters act as a balancer and are useful for inducing a sense of relaxation and lifting the mood, making petitgrain a good oil for women with mood swings, stress and anxiety. It can help insomnia and restlessness, possibly by easing respiration and relaxing the muscles (Sellar 1992, p. 129). It seems to have a soothing action on the emotions, especially in cases of panic, and could be useful for the transition stage of labour. The author has used petitgrain to treat antenatal women with anxiety, as well as those with postpartum 'blues' or depression; there appears to be a powerful synergistic effect when used in conjunction with jasmine and/or neroli.

Several alcohols are found in the oil including linalol, nerol, geraniol, terpineol, farnesol, nerolidol and citronellol, and these together with the esters and the terpenes, limonene and camphene, give the oil antibacterial, antifungal, antiviral and general antiseptic properties. It has been used for acne and other skin disorders and may be a suitable oil for women who develop a greasy skin during pregnancy, administered as a facial sauna. It can also be added to the rinsing water for greasy hair and may help when a pregnant woman perspires excessively due to the physiological rise in temperature.

A small proportion of the aldehyde citral assists in the anti-infective qualities and, with the alcohols, acts as a hypotensive and temperature-reducing agent.

As with many other of the citrus essences, petitgrain can be effective in treating constipation, flatulence and indigestion, an action that is probably enhanced when blending a synergistic mix of petitgrain and orange, mandarin or neroli.

Dangers   Petitgrain oil is thought to be non-toxic, non-irritant and non-sensitizing, although this latter is contentious as a small number of subjects with existing dermatological conditions have been found to become sensitive to it and it is recommended that very low dilutions are used for these clients (International School of Aromatherapy 1993, p. 65).

Blends   Petitgrain blends well with other citrus oils such as bergamot, grapefruit, mandarin, neroli and sweet orange as well as with benzoin, citronella, clary sage, geranium, lavender, jasmine, rosemary, rosewood, sandalwood and ylang ylang.

Rose – *Rosa damascena, centifolia* and *gallica* (Rosaceae family)

Rose oil is among the most luxurious in the world and, together with jasmine and neroli, is one of the most expensive. Although there are several hundred species and hybrids of rose, only three main species are used for essential oil production as these are the most aromatic. *Rosa damascena*, grown in Bulgaria, is steam distilled then decanted to separate the oil from the water and so produce rose otto or attar; a rose absolute is produced through solvent extraction (previously through enfleurage) from *R. centifolia* in France; more commonly nowadays a hybrid of *R. centifolia* and *R. gallica*, called rose de mai, is grown to produce an absolute or concrete (Lawless 1992, p. 157). Roses are extremely sensitive to climatic changes and some crops produce oils of superior quality while others are not so good. The absolutes are not generally used for therapeutic work as essential oils are steam distilled from the original extract and are more suited to aromatherapy.

When buying rose essential oil it is wise to be guided by price to a certain extent, for it takes the petals of approximately 60 000 roses to produce one ounce of the oil (Tisserand 1992, p. 272).

Roses and their aroma are pleasing to almost everyone, and such is the plant's popularity that a Rose Museum has been established near Frankfurt, the only one of its kind in the world, devoted to collecting, exhibiting and researching this marvellous flower (Kubler & Wabner 1994).

Chemical constituents   The chemical constituents of the different types of rose oil are similar, although the balance of these chemicals may vary significantly depending on soil, weather, geography and the method of extraction. There are over 300 constituents of rose which have been identified, even though some of them are in negligible amounts. However, Brud & Konopacka–Brud (1994) suggest that the aroma and the therapeutic properties may depend on the ratios of these minor constituents.

Citronellol (around 20%) and phenyl ethanol (up to 60%), eugenol, farnesol, geraniol, linalol and nerol, which are alcohols, are present in varying amounts and contribute towards the anti–infective and immunostimulant properties of rose oil. The vasoconstrictive and astringent actions of the alcohols help in controlling haemostasis, and rose oil can be effective for a variety of skin conditions.

The rose seems to have a great affinity with the female reproductive tract and, with its lovely feminine aroma, is particularly suited to use in maternity and gynaecological care. Rose oil may be used to regulate the menstrual cycle, for premenstrual tension and the menopause, menorrhagia, dysmenorrhoea, leucorrhoea and post-hysterectomy syndrome. In labour it can be very relaxing and can aid uterine action. However, while Tisserand & Balacs (1995, p. 111) disagree that its emmenagogic actions preclude its use during pregnancy, it would be wise to be cautious and avoid administration until late pregnancy. Postnatally it can be a lovely addition to a massage or a bath oil, perhaps combined with jasmine for a real luxury.

Digestive and hepatic conditions can be treated, such as biliary nausea, constipation and even cholecystitis, according to Lawless (1992, p. 159). Holmes (1994) attributes this to the cooling, drying nature of the oil, as defined in Chinese and traditional Greek medicine. Kirov et al (1988a) tested rose oil on rats and found it to have a hepato-protective action. Further work by Kirov et al (1988b) examined the toxic effects of oral administration of rose oil to rats and concluded that the appropriate therapeutic dose for humans, if used, as postulated, to treat atherosclerosis, would be 2–4 mg/kg daily, orally. This far exceeds the dose that would be used for dermal application in clinical aromatherapy.

However, the main value of rose oil is in relieving stress-related conditions, including tension, insomnia and depression, possibly as a result of the balancing action of the oil's effect on the hypothalamus (Holmes (1994) quotes nearly 30 emotions that may respond to rose oil). The relaxing and aphrodisiac qualities can be helpful for frigidity and impotence caused by emotional factors, and may trigger the release of dopamine from the brain (Sellar 1992, p. 135). Tasev et al (1969) found that rose stimulated neuro-psychic activity by increasing concentration and attention spans and decreasing response times. This was echoed by Sugano & Sato (1991). Conversely rose oil was found to suppress cardiac response patterns (Kikuchi et al 1991).

Dangers   It is vital, when purchasing rose oil, to ensure it is of the highest possible quality, although this can be confirmed only by chromatography. (Reputable suppliers may provide a printout of the analysis.) A variety of synthetic chemicals may be used to adulterate the oil, or additions of other oils that smell similar and contain similar chemical constituents, such as rose geranium, may be found in the retailed product.

When an absolute is produced, chemical solvents are used, traces of which may be found in the final extract. This is important as most of the readily available rose oil will be an absolute, for up to six times more absolute can be extracted than essential oil (Holmes 1994).

Blends   Rose is classed as having a middle to base note, from a perfumery point of view, and tends to be a subtle addition to a blend, with the main strength of the aroma becoming evident after it has warmed. It blends well with benzoin, bergamot, camomile, cedarwood, clary sage, geranium, grapefruit, jasmine, lavender, lemon, lime, mandarin, melissa, neroli, sweet orange, patchouli, rosewood, sandalwood, tangerine and ylang ylang.

Rosemary – *Rosmarinus officinalis* (Labiatae family)

This oil has a strong herbal and quite penetrating camphorous aroma and has a long tradition of medicinal usage. It is steam distilled from the flowers and leaves, but a poorer quality oil is also obtained from the whole plant, primarily in Spain (Plate 6).

Chemical constituents   As might be expected from the aroma, rosemary contains a small amount of camphor, which is a ketone, and another of this group, thujone, making the oil potentially abortifacient and therefore should be *used with great caution* in pregnancy, although it could be used in small doses near term. Indeed, Tisserand & Balacs (1995, p. 111) suggest that rosemary is safe to use externally, in massage, but should not be admin-istered internally or via mucous membranes during pregnancy. The ketones, together with almost 50% of the oxide 1,8-cineole, account for the expectorant, decongestant and mucolytic properties, so that rosemary can be extremely effective in clearing the head in people with colds and influenza.

The cephalic effects (stimulating and energizing the mind) have long been known, and indeed Shakespeare's 'rosemary for remembrance' helps to remind us of one of the uses for this oil. Kovar et al (1987) demonstrated the stimulating effects of oil of rosemary in mice, although they were not able to attribute this effect to any individual component. Midwives on night duty could consider putting two drops on a handkerchief to sniff in order to keep them alert and awake! Postnatally rosemary could be given to an exhausted mother as a temporary relief, especially if she has tension headaches or mild 'blues'.

Monoterpenes and sesquiterpenes in the form of camphene, limonene, pinene and β-caryophyllene contribute to the analgesic action, which is particularly effective for muscular aches and pains and could be useful for women in labour or for dysmenorrhoea. Premenstrually and postnatally it may help to reduce oedema.

Various alcohols (borneol, terpineol and linalol) assist in the generally anti-infective value of the essential oil, and the stimulating and uplifting actions. A partial antimicrobial action was demonstrated by Soliman et al (1994), who found the oil effective against *Mycobacterium intracellulare, Candida albicans* and *Cryptococcus neoformans* but not against *Staphylococcus aureus, Escherichia coli, Pseudomonas aeruginosa* and others.

Similar limited antibacterial activity was found by Boatto et al (1994), although the antifungal activity against *Candida albicans* was found to be greater in rosemary than in sage oil (Steinmetz et al 1988). Pandit & Shelef (1994) suggest that the inhibitory effect of rosemary on *Listeria monocytogenes* may be due to the antioxidant components, carnisol and ursolic acid. Recent research (Domokos et al 1997) indicates that a newly developed, frost-resistant Hungarian rosemary plant produces an essential oil different in composition from other rosemary oils, and that it inhibits 50% more Gram-negative bacteria than other commercially available rosemary oils.

The alcohols are responsible for a vasoconstrictive effect and it is probably for this reason that rosemary is a hypertensive oil: it may be beneficial for women with hypotension but should be avoided in those with raised blood pressure although Tisserand & Balacs (1995, p. 65) query whether rosemary is in fact *hypotensive*. They state that, as there is no evidence of the effect of essential oils on human blood pressure, there are no contraindications to the use of essential oils for people with hyper- or hypotension, by any route. The astringency contributes to wound healing, and interestingly Tisserand (1992, p. 281) states that the Arabs apply the powdered herb, as an antiseptic and haemostatic, to the umbilical cords of newborn babies.

Rosemary is a component of many proprietary hair-care products and the oil can be added to rinsing water for greasy hair, and used in a variety of scalp and hair disorders such as dandruff, seborrhoea and thinning hair – helpful for women whose hair thins during pregnancy or, more often, in the months following delivery.

A small amount of the antispasmodic ester bornyl acetate helps gastro-intestinal discomforts such as flatulence, colic (but best avoided in babies), dyspepsia and possibly gallbladder problems. This spasmolytic activity is thought to be a result of acetylcholine antagonism (Aqel 1991, Taddei et al 1988). Al-Hader et al (1994) also found that rosemary oil increased blood glucose and decreased insulin levels in rabbits.

Dangers   Rosemary essential oil *should be used sparingly during pregnancy.* It may be wise to restrict its use in women with deviations from normal blood pressure. It should not be used by epileptics, although very small amounts may work homoeopathically to treat epilepsy (Davis 1988, p. 293).

Adulteration with turpentine oils or another essential oil such as sage may occur, so careful purchasing is necessary to ensure purity. Svoboda & Deans (1990) examined 10 samples of essential oil of rosemary which showed a wide range of proportions of the varying constituents. It was stated that camphor or eucalyptus oils were frequently used to adulterate the rosemary oil. The strong aroma may antidote homoeopathic remedies.

Blends   Rosemary's strong camphorous aroma blends well with basil, cedarwood, frankincense, geranium, ginger, grapefruit, lavender, lime, mandarin, melissa, orange, petitgrain, tangerine and thyme.

Rosewood – *Aniba rosaeodora* (Lauraceae family)   This essential oil, extracted by steam distillation from the wood chippings, has only recently come into use in aromatherapy, although its continued use is in doubt, for the trees originate in the Brazilian rain forests and are being extensively felled for wood. Practitioners concerned about environmental issues should be aware that its production is reputed to be contributing to the damage resulting from deforestation, and they may therefore wish to refrain from its use. However, rosewood oil is also available from Peru and Guyana and, although the crop is smaller and there are logistical problems of transportation which increase the price, rosewood oil from these countries does not interfere with the environment. Additionally the harvesting is controlled and replanting is actively encouraged (Aqua Oleum 1993).

Chemical constituents   One of the main constituents is the alcohol, linalol (about 80–97% according to its country of origin), with geraniol, nerol and terpineol. These, and the terpenes, limonene, pinene and terpinene, mean that the oil has anti-infective properties, immunostimulant action (due to the alcohols) and some mild analgesic effects (terpenes).

The alcohols and a small amount of the aldehyde citronellal make it relaxing, mood uplifting and hypotensive, although it may also have a stimulating action and is therefore considered to be a balancer. It is of value as an aphrodisiac, anti-stress remedy and for nervous tension symptoms such as headache and nausea. McArdle (1992) reported its benefits in reducing blood pressure in a woman with fulminating pre-eclampsia, although this may have been due in part to the method of administration.

Skin conditions seem to respond fairly well to rosewood and it may have a part to play in wound healing, prevention of striae gravidarum and even ageing skin.

Dangers   Some aromatherapists believe that rosewood can be substituted with Ho wood oil as the linalol content is similar, but this is not appropriate for the balance of other constituents will be different; Price (1993, p. 114) suggests experimenting with Ho wood (*Cinnamomum camphora*) for its *similar aroma* or even with rhodium wood oil (*Convolvulus scoparius*, often referred to as 'rosewood', and usually found as a blend of geranium or palmarosa combined with sandalwood). While, in principle, Price may have a point in that these alternatives may achieve the desired therapeutic effects without using true rosewood oil, it seems somewhat irresponsible to advise these substitutions for clinical work. Furthermore it again emphasizes the need for aromatherapists to adopt the practice of referring to oils by their Latin names rather than their common names so that the correct, most appropriate, oil may be selected. It is not good practice either to use a synthetic form of linalol for therapeutic work, and midwives and aromatherapists should ensure that they purchase their *Aniba rosaeodora* from a reputable supplier and not from a perfume source.

Blends   Rosewood blends well with cajuput, cedarwood, frankincense, geranium, grapefruit, jasmine, mandarin, marjoram, orange, patchouli, petitgrain, rose, rosemary, sandalwood, tangerine and ylang ylang.

Sandalwood – *Santalum album* (Santalaceae family)

Most commercially available sandalwood oil comes from trees grown in the Mysore region of India, all of which are now owned and controlled by the Indian government as a conservationary measure, although, until the replanting process results in more established trees, this has served only to increase the price artificially. Consequently many buyers of sandalwood oil have turned to Indonesia and China, and some oil comes from New Caledonia but is very expensive owing to transportation costs.

Another type of sandalwood (*Eurcarya spicata* or *Santalum spicatum*) is grown in Australia and, although this is a very effective agent against Gram-positive bacteria, *Staphylococcus aureus* and *Candida albicans*, it is currently a protected species and therefore the oil is not available commercially (International School of Aromatherapy 1993, p. 63). Sandalwood oil is extracted by steam distillation from wood chips from the inner heartwood and the roots, and allowed to mature for up to 6 months, when it is re-distilled under vacuum to produce an oil suitable for use, the initial distillate being too crude.

Chemical constituents   The main constituent is a mixture of two sesqui-terpenic alcohols, called santalol (around 90%). Other alcohols such as borneol and teresantol, approximately 6% santalene and other sesquiter-penes, and the aldehyde furfurol are also present. Jirovetz et al's (1992) investigations in which blood samples from mice that had inhaled sandalwood oil were analysed, showed α-santalol, β-santalol and α-santalene to be present in significant amounts; when given pure fragrance compounds, the blood analyses also showed the presence of coumarins and α-terpineol.

The oil's principal value lies in its affinity with the genitourinary and respiratory systems, and with the gastrointestinal tract. Anecdotal evidence suggests that sandalwood is extremely effective in combating cystitis and urinary tract infections, as well as genital discharges, for example leucor-rhoea and the urethral/vaginal discharge in gonorrhoea. Massage of the oil into the suprapubic and sacral areas has an anti-inflammatory and anti-infective effect, and is generally soothing. In the case of gonorrhoea, Tisserand (1992, p. 284) surmises that sandalwood's action is not due directly to an antibacterial effect, but that it 'abolishes spontaneous con-tractions of the spermatic cord, lessens the motility of the genital tract muscles, has a diuretic effect and inhibits secretions', although there does not appear to be any evidence for this sweeping claim.

Expectoration and reduction in sputum production can be achieved by administering sandalwood as an inhalation; it can be of benefit for bron-chitis, coughs, colds, catarrh and sore throats, partly through the mucolytic and decongestant actions but also due to the antiseptic property. A facial sauna can effectively treat acne and greasy skin.

Sandalwood is a very relaxing oil, which may account for its well-known aphrodisiac quality. Okugawa et al (1995) found the α- and β-san-talol constituents to be responsible for the neuroleptic, sedative (but not anticonvulsant) effects. Certainly the aroma is pleasing to both men and women, and it may be of assistance in treating puerperal frigidity or impo-tence when there is an underlying psychological cause. The astringency of sandalwood may help in combating diarrhoea, and it has been used to good effect for nausea and vomiting and for heartburn.

Dangers   The prohibitive cost and limited availability of pure, legal, sandalwood oil often leads to its adulteration with other oils such as palm, linseed or castor, or with essential oils, e.g. guaiacwood or cedarwood. Those who are concerned should enquire from their supplier as to the quality and source of the oil.

Sellar (1992, p. 143) suggests that the potency of the relaxation effect of the oil precludes its use in people who are pathologically depressed as it may lower their mood even further, making them completely introspective.

Although Tisserand & Balacs (1995, p. 82) surmise that there is a neg-ligible risk of dermal irritation, Sharma et al (1987) report the case of sen-sitivity to sandalwood oil, but this was following a protracted period of application of sandalwood paste.

Blends   Sandalwood's aroma is a base note and it lingers for a considerable length of time after use. The oil blends well with basil, benzoin, black pepper, clary sage, cypress, frankincense, geranium, jasmine, juniper berry, lavender, lemon, mandarin, neroli, orange, patchouli, petitgrain, rose, rosewood and ylang ylang.

Tea or ti tree –
Melaleuca
alternifolia
(Myrtaceae family)

Tea tree is indigenous to Australia and has long been part of Aboriginal medicine. The oil was introduced to Europe in the early 1920s and used for its antiseptic qualities, particularly in the Second World War. The leaves and branches from which the oil is steam distilled have to be gathered by hand for the tree grows in snake-infested swampground and machine harvesting would be difficult. The yield from crops harvested in the Australian summer months from November to February is greater than that in the winter, but climatic conditions and the threat of bush fires may affect the crop. The massive worldwide increase in interest in the therapeutic properties of tea tree, especially among the medical profession, means that demand is overtaking supply and, although currently not an expensive essential oil, it is likely that the price will rise considerably in the not-too-distant future. The Australia Tea Tree Management Limited has helped with the breeding of *Melaleuca alternifolia* and other varieties of tea tree, including *Melaleuca linariifolia*, which has high levels of terpinen-4-ol (Williams et al 1998).

Chemical constituents   Alcohols and terpenes form the main constituents of tea tree oil. A large amount of the alcohol terpinen-4-ol with smaller amounts of α-terpineol and linalol, together with the monoterpenes, *d*-limonene, myrcene, phellandrene and pinene, and the sesquiterpenes, α-terpinene, γ-terpinene, sabinene and β-caryophyllene, combine to make the oil a powerful antiseptic, antibacterial, antiviral, antifungal and antimicrobial agent. Altman (1989) found that tea tree was 11 times more effective as a disinfectant and antiseptic than phenols, and Pena's early (1962) investigations showed its effectiveness in treating trichomonal and candidal infections of the vagina by means of tampons and douches. Likewise, Belaiche (1985a) demonstrated its action against *Candida albicans*, while Carson & Riley (1994) found that tea tree inhibited the actions not only of *C. albicans*, but also of *Escherichia coli, Staphylococcus aureus, Bacteroides fragilis, Mycobacterium smegmatis* and *Clostridium perfringens*. Belaiche (1985b) also used tea tree oil to treat skin infections such as staphylococcal acne, staphylococcal and streptococcal impetigo and *C. albicans*. Carson & Riley (1995) have explored the value of *Melaleuca* in tackling methicillin-resistant *S. aureus* and cite similar work by researchers in the UK. Williams et al (1998) also comment on this potential use and cite Sweet (1997) and others. Zarno (1994) recommends tea tree as the oil of first choice for candidiasis, and it can be administered in proprietary pessary form or on tampons soaked in tea tree solution for women with vaginal thrush.

Bassett et al (1990) compared tea tree oil and benzoyl peroxide in the treatment of acne and found that, although the tea tree acted more slowly, it was equally as effective as the benzoyl peroxide but with fewer side effects. This was similar to findings by Tong et al (1992) in respect of the treatment of tinea pedis. Raman et al (1995) and Carson & Riley (1994) also found tea tree oil to be effective in alleviating acne, and women who develop this condition during pregnancy could use facial saunas of tea tree oil or add a few drops to cooled, boiled water to use when washing. Hammer et al (1996) demonstrated the effectiveness of tea tree oil in removing transient skin flora while maintaining those which were resident, which may indicate its value as a preventative agent when added to bathwater for women about to undergo planned Caesarean section and afterwards.

There is much contemporary work into the use of tea tree oil as an anti-infective agent, with the principal active ingredient being identified as terpinen-4-ol (Carson & Riley 1995, Carson et al 1996, Watt, personal communication 1996, Williams et al 1998). Southwell et al (1997) questioned whether tea tree oils with a high level of 1,8-cineole would reduce the anti-infective properties of the total oils, and found that those with levels higher than 15% had a corresponding decrease in the percentage of terpinen-4-ol, thereby rendering it less effective. Williams et al (1998) state that there is now an Australian standard for good quality tea tree oil for clinical purposes which requires the oil to have a 1,8-cineole level of less than 15% and a terpinen-4-ol content of more than 30%. Practitioners should, therefore, insist that the tea tree oil they are buying has a sufficiently high proportion of terpinen-4-ol.

Australian and New Zealand plant oils as medicinal products are increasingly being tested for antimicrobial activity and there is some suggestion that the relatively newly discovered oils of manuka and kanuka may be as efficient as tea tree (Cooke & Cooke 1991), although Lis-Balchin et al (1996a) suggest that there is no justification for their use, when other oils that are equally effective, such as tea tree, are available. Dilute additions of tea tree oil to the bath or bidet may assist in preventing or treating infection of the perineum following suturing. Compresses applied suprapubically or sacrally may relieve cystitis and urinary tract infection. Inhalations of tea tree could be offered to women at risk of developing chest infection after surgery and would be a more natural means of treating colds and influenza in pregnancy, when drugs are contraindicated. Extremely small doses could be added to a barrier cream in the event of napkin rash in the baby, although this should probably not be used preventatively owing to the risk of dermal irritation (see below).

Dangers   Tea tree oil appears to be non-toxic and non-irritant. However, although it has been used successfully to treat skin disorders, it has also been reported to cause dermatitis in some individuals, particularly after prolonged application (DeGroot 1996, De Groot & Weyland 1993, Knight & Hausen 1994, Selvaag et al 1994, Southwell et al 1997). In Knight & Hausen's research the eczema and vesiculation that occurred in seven patients was most commonly found to be an allergy to *d*-limonene, with some allergy to α-terpinene and terpinen-4-ol.

Beccara (1995) reports the case of a toddler who ingested less than 10 ml of *Melaleuca alternifolia*. Fortunately, after treatment, he recovered and there is no evidence of the effects of ingesting large amounts of the oil; it would seem that the lesson learnt from this case is less about tea tree oil specifically, and more to do with the storage of essential oils generally.

Blends Tea tree oil has a strong medicinal aroma which blends well with cinnamon, cypress, eucalyptus, ginger, lavender, lemon, lemongrass, mandarin, marjoram, nutmeg, orange, rosemary, tangerine and thyme.

Ylang ylang –
Cananga odorata
(Anonaceae family)

Ylang ylang essential oil is produced from the flowers of the tree, but there are several different grades obtained and only the purest should be used in therapeutic aromatherapy. It has a sweet floral and very heady aroma which can make some people feel nauseated.

Chemical constituents Linalol (up to 30%), geraniol and farnesol (alcohols) contribute towards the reputation of ylang ylang as an antidepressant and general tonic, while the ester benzyl acetate and the phenols eugenol and safrole aid its sedative action. The monoterpene pinene and the sesquiterpene cadinene, together with the phenols, assist in the antiseptic and antibacterial properties, which seem particularly effective with gastrointestinal infections. The alcohols and the cadinene are hypotensive.

Ylang ylang is renowned as a treatment for emotionally related conditions such as stress, panic, anxiety, sexual problems and hypertension. It appears to be safe to use in pregnancy in small doses and can help women who are very nervous and worried about their approaching labour.

Dangers The high price of the superior grades of ylang ylang oil mean that it is open to adulteration with the inferior Cananga oil or other additions such as coconut oil. Ryman (1991, p. 218) suggests standing the bottle of oil in the refrigerator for a short while; if it is adulterated, it will thicken and become cloudy.

The aroma can be overpowering for some clients and it should be used in small doses intermittently; prolonged use may be stimulating rather than relaxing.

Blends Ylang ylang blends well with lighter oils, which can subdue its intensity. These include bergamot, black pepper, camomile, grapefruit, jasmine, lavender, lemon, lime, marjoram, melissa, neroli, orange, patchouli, petitgrain, rose, rosewood and sandalwood.

Carrier or base oils

Essential oils are highly concentrated and, with only a very few exceptions, should rarely be used neat on the skin. This applies equally to using the oils in a massage blend or in the bath. The essential oils should be diluted into a good quality vegetable oil; mineral oils are not used as they do not allow the essential oil to absorb into the skin adequately, and may also contain lanolin, to which some people are allergic.

The carrier oil serves as a lubricant when performing massage, enabling the hands of the practitioner to glide over the skin surface smoothly without friction. Different carrier oils are used for different purposes, but common to all is the need for the carrier to be 100% pure and without an odour that could overpower the aromas of the essential oils.

Most carrier oils contain vitamins and minerals, and the texture will moisturize the skin. They may be produced from the nuts, seeds, beans or kernels of a variety of plants.

The following carrier oils are a few of the more commonly used oils, although there is a wide range of different ones from which to choose.

Almond, sweet – *Prunus amygdalis*

Sweet almond oil is derived from the kernels of the almonds by warm pressing; it should not be confused with the bitter almond, the oil of which may contain prussic acid or cyanide (hydrocyanic acid) produced during the extraction process. Sweet almond trees have pink blossom, whereas bitter almond trees have white blossom. The oil is usually pale yellow, although the colour can vary according to the time of harvesting, from a greenish tinge to a deep gold. Completely colourless sweet almond oil is likely to have been refined and will no longer contain the vitamins A, B_1, B_2, B_6 and E, or the minerals and the monounsaturated and polyunsaturated fatty acids present in unrefined almond oil.

Sweet almond is one of the most popular carrier oils used in aromatherapy and is not overly expensive; the vitamin E content helps to preserve the oil. It is slightly sticky in texture and can be used on its own or mixed with another carrier oil. It will nourish the skin and is thought to be useful in cases of eczema and other irritations.

Concern regarding the potential for the development of nut allergies in babies born to women who have eaten nuts, may prompt practitioners to consider restraint in the use of sweet almond carrier oil in pregnancy, although there is no evidence to support this belief.

Apricot kernel – *Prunus armeniaca*

Apricot oil is extracted from the seed kernels and is high in essential fatty acids, although, unlike the fruit, it does not contain many vitamins. The oil is light in texture, particularly suited to facial massage, and to dry, sensitive or mature skins as it is absorbed easily.

Avocado – *Persea americana*

Mechanical pressing followed by centrifugal extraction is used to obtain avocado oil from the flesh of the fruit, grown largely in Mexico and in other parts of the southern United States and South America. The unrefined oil is a deep green colour and full of vitamins, lecithin, protein and essential fatty acids. It has a tendency to become cloudy and thick and, when cold, to solidify (although gentle warming of the bottle with the hands will reverse this process), leading producers in the cosmetics industry to refine the oil, which is then not suitable for use in aromatherapy.

The thick consistency and expensive price of avocado oil usually result in practitioners blending it with another carrier such as almond or grapeseed oil, but this does enhance the skin-nourishing properties of the final blend.

Avocado oil may be a pleasant addition to a blend to be used for abdominal massage in pregnancy, possibly helping to prevent striae gravidarum.

Grapeseed – *Vitis vinferi*

This oil is obtained from the seeds of grapes, often imported from wine-growing areas in Europe. It is a yellow-green colour and very light in texture, without any noticeable odour. Grapeseed is universally used in aromatherapy for its non-greasy, silky feeling and because it is inexpensive, even more so than sweet almond oil. However, most grapeseed oils available on the market have been refined and lack the original nutrients, so it is wise to mix it with another, more nourishing, carrier for best effects.

Peach kernel – *Prunus persica*

Peach kernel oil is similar to apricot kernel and is high in monounsaturates and polyunsaturates and vitamin E, making it good for facial massage. This is especially so as it is thought to stimulate secretion of the body's own naturally occurring oils and to encourage skin suppleness and elasticity; this could also be beneficial for abdominal massage in pregnancy.

Sesame seed – *Sesamum indicum*

The oil is extracted from the seeds, which can yield up to 60% pure oil. It is light and has virtually no odour, and has the advantage of washing out of towels better than grapeseed or sweet almond oil. As it is a monounsaturated oil it will retain its freshness longer than some other oils and will not go rancid in strong sunlight or excessive heat. Indeed, sesame oil can act as a fairly good sunfilter and is about 10% more effective than many other carriers.

The oil can be used as a carrier on its own or mixed with another, and moisturizes dry skin.

Wheatgerm – *Triticum vulgare*

Cold expression of the wheatgerm is performed to extract this dark orange-brown oil which is thick, rich and very nourishing, containing vitamin E and essential fatty acids. The vitamin E makes wheatgerm oil a natural antioxidant, i.e. it helps to prevent the deterioration that may occur when the oil is exposed to oxygen, light or temperature changes. Adding a small proportion (10–25%) of wheatgerm to another base oil will enrich it, making it useful for dry skins or scar tissue and burns, and will prolong the 'shelf-life' of a carrier into which has been added essential oils.

There are many other carrier oils, but those outlined above are easily available, in the main relatively inexpensive and offer a versatile selection for the purposes of aromatherapy. Other base oils include borage, calendula, carrot, evening primrose, hazelnut, jojoba and macadamia nut oil.

Essential Oils Suitable for Pregnancy and Childbirth

Essential oil	Uses in childbirth	Precautions
Basil	Pain relief in labour Chest infections, sinus congestion Retained placenta Postnatal 'blues'	Pregnancy Sensitive skin High doses
Benzoin	Cystitis Colic, flatulence, constipation Coughs, colds, sore throats Wound healing Stress, tension, anxiety	Sensitive skin
Bergamot	Cystitis, urinary tract infection Indigestion, colic, flatulence Viral infections Acne Pain relief in labour	Sunbathing
Black pepper	Pain relief in labour Bruising Constipation	Renal disease Women on diuretics Sensitive skin
Camomile	Cystitis, urinary tract infections Ophthalmia neonatorum Wound healing, sore nipples Pain relief in labour Backache, headache, afterpains Inducing rest and sleep	Sensitive skin
Clary sage	Respiratory infections Pain relief in labour Stress, depression	Pregnancy Care if driving Potentiates alcohol

Eucalyptus	Respiratory infections Cystitis	Sensitive skin Ingestion Epilepsy Hypertension With homoeopathy
Frankincense	Respiratory infections Urinary tract infections Anxiety in labour or postnatally	
Geranium	Oedema Pain relief in labour Sore nipples or perineum	Ensure purity
Ginger	Nausea and vomiting Diarrhoea, flatulence	Sensitive skin Sunlight
Grapefruit	Depression, stress, anxiety Nausea and vomiting, pica	Citrus allergy Store in refrigerator
Jasmine	Pain relief in labour Postnatal depression	Pregnancy Ensure purity
Juniper berry	Postnatal oedema	Pregnancy? History of renal disease Hypertension
Lavender	Pain relief in labour Headache Poor uterine action Wound healing	Hypotension Epidural anaesthesia Early pregnancy
Lemon	Infections Anaemia? Hypertension Gastric acidity	Sensitive skin
Lemongrass	Infections Pain relief in labour Inadequate lactation Heartburn, flatulence Loss of appetite	Sensitive skin
Lime	Depression, anxiety Loss of appetite, pica	Sunlight
Mandarin	Constipation Aids relaxation	Citrus allergy
Marjoram	Constipation, colic Pain relief in labour Colds, influenza	Early pregnancy

Neroli	Stress, anxiety, depression Poor uterine action Reduced libido postnatally Insomnia	Care if driving
Nutmeg	Digestive complaints Pain relief in labour	*Never* in pregnancy
Orange	Hypertension Insomina, stress Nausea and vomiting Constipation, colic Oedema	Citrus allergy
Patchouli	Poor libido Wound healing	Quality (?adulteration)
Petitgrain	Mood swings, stress Transition in labour Gastric discomfort	Skin sensitivity
Rose	Enhance contractions Depression, insomnia	Pregnancy
Rosemary	Stimulation, aids concentration Pain in labour Hypotension Hair care	Early pregnancy Hypertension? Epilepsy
Rosewood	Hypertension, pre-eclampsia Mood enhancer, relaxant	Purity
Sandalwood	Cystitis, urinary tract infections Genital infection Respiratory infections Poor libido	Purity Clinical depression
Tea tree	Vaginal infections Wound infections Respiratory infections	Skin irritation
Ylang ylang	Relaxation, stress Hypertension Antidepressant	Purity

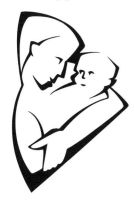

Appendix 2 **Glossary of Terms and Properties of Essential Oils**

Analgesic	pain relieving
Antacid	combats acidity
Antibiotic	combats bacterial infection
Anticoagulant	prevents blood clotting
Antidepressant	relieves depression
Antidontalgic	relieves toothache
Antiemetic	combats nausea and vomiting
Antimicrobial	fights microbial infection
Antiphlogistic	reduces inflammation
Antiseptic	controls infection
Antispasmodic	relieves cramp
Antisudorific	reduces sweating
Antiviral	fights viral infection
Aperitif	stimulates appetite
Aphrodisiac	increases sexual desire
Astringent	tightens and binds tissues
Balsamic	reduces and softens mucus
Bechic	eases coughing
Cardiac	stimulates heart
Carminative	encourages expulsion of flatus
Cephalic	stimulates, clears the mind
Cholagogue	increases bile secretion
Cicatrisant	helps formation of scar tissue
Cytoprophylactic	encourages growth of new cells
Decongestant	reduces mucus production
Deodorant	destroys odour
Depurative	purifies the blood
Digestive	aids digestion
Diuretic	stimulates micturition

Emmenagogue	induces uterine bleeding
Expectorant	clears excess mucus from bronchioles
Febrifuge	reduces pyrexia
Fungicide	fights fungal infections
Galactagogue	encourages lactation
Haemostatic	stops haemorrhage
Hepatic	stimulates liver and gallbladder
Hypertensive	increases blood pressure
Hypotensive	lowers blood pressure
Laxative	encourages bowel movements
Parturient	eases labour and delivery
Rubefacient	increases circulation, warming
Sedative	calming
Stimulant	increases energy and adrenaline
Stomachic	relieves gastric disorders
Sudorific	increases sweating
Uterine	tonic for the uterus
Vasoconstrictor	contracts blood vessel walls
Vasodilator	dilates blood vessel walls

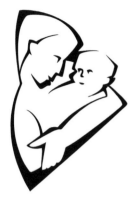

Appendix 3 **Useful Addresses**

Aromatherapy Database
c/o Bob Harris
2 Ruelle du Tertre
St Germain le Guillaume
Bûtet 53240
France

Offers literature-searching facility for essential oil research

Aromatherapy Organizations Council
PO Box 19824
London
SE 25 6WF
Tel: 0208 251 7912

British Complementary Medicine Association
249 Fosse Road South
Leicester
LE3 1AE
Tel: 0116 282 5511

Holds registers of complementary therapy organizations.

British School of Reflex Zone Therapy
23 Marsh Hall
Talisman Way
Wembley Park
Middlesex
HA9 8JJ
Tel: 020 8904 4825

British Shiatsu Council
121 Sheen Road
Richmond
Surrey
TW9 1YS
Tel: 020 8852 1080

Complementary Therapies in Maternity Care National Forum
c/o Denise Tiran (Chair)
School of Health
University of Greenwich
Grey, Southwood Site
Avery Hill Campus
Avery Hill Road
Eltham
London SE9 2UG
Tel: 020 8331 8000

Multidisciplinary networking and support forum for all professionals interested in integrating complementary therapies into conventional maternity care

Institute for Complementary Medicine
PO Box 194
London SE16 1QZ
Tel: 020 7237 5165

Holds register of individual practitioners of complementary medicine: good-sized library

International Journal of Aromatherapy
PO Box 746
Hove
East Sussex
BN3 2BD
Tel: 01273 772479

Research Council for Complementary Medicine
60 Great Ormond Street
London WC1N 3JF
Tel: 020 7833 8897

Offers literature searches on complementary medicine; access to many international databases

Talking Pictures
 PO Box 77
Cirencester
Gloucestershire GL7 5YN
www.talkingpictures.co.uk
Video 'A Practical Guide to Childbirth Massage Techniques', price £15.95

University of Greenwich, School of Health
Honeycombe Building, Mansion Site
Avery Hill Campus
Avery Hill Road
Eltham
London SE9 2UG
Tel 020 8331 8000

Offers BSc(Hons) degree in Complementary Therapies with a generic route plus specialisms in aromatherapy and stress management

References and Further Reading

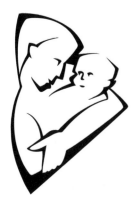

References

Abdel Wahab S M, Aboutel E A, Wl-Zalabani S M et al 1987 The essential oil of olibanum. Planta Medica 3:382–384

Aboutabl E A, Abdelhakim G 1996 A study of some pharmacodynamic actions of certain *Melaleuca* species grown in Egypt. Phytotherapy Research 10:345–347

Abraham M, Devi N S, Sheela R 1979 Inhibiting effect of jasmine flowers on lactation. Indian Journal of Medical Research 69:88–92

Achterrath-Tuckermann U, Kunde R, Flaskamp E et al 1980 Pharmacological investigations with compounds of chamomile. Investigations on the spasmolytic effects of compounds of chamomile and Kamillosan on the isolated guinea pig ileum. Planta Medica 39:38–50

Acolet D, Modi N, Giannakoulopoulos X et al 1993 Changes in plasma cortisol and catecholamine concentrations in response to massage in preterm infants. Archives of Disease in Childhood (Fetal and Neonatal Edition) 68(1):29–31

Adamson S 1996a Teaching baby massage to new parents. Complementary Therapies in Nursing and Midwifery 2(6):151–159

Adamson S 1996b Hands-on therapy. Health Visitor 66(2):48–50

Adamson-Macedo E N, Dattani I, Wilson A et al 1993 Small sample follow-up study of children who received tactile stimulation after pre-term birth: intelligence and achievements. Journal of Reproductive and Infant Psychology 11(3):165–168

Adamson-Macedo E N, de Roiste A, Wilson A et al 1994a TAC-TIC therapy with high-risk distressed ventilated preterms. Journal of

Reproductive and Infant Psychology 12(4):249–252

Adamson-Macedo E N, Attree J L A et al 1994b TAC-TIC therapy: the importance of systematic stroking. British Journal of Midwifery 2(6):264, 266–269

Adamson-Macedo E N, de Roiste A, Wilson A et al 1997 Systematic gentle/light stroking and maternal random touching of ventilated preterm: a preliminary study. International Journal of Prenatal and Perinatal Psychology and Medicine 9(1):17–31

Aertgeerts P, Abring M, Klaschka F et al 1985 Comparative testing of Kamillosan cream and steroidal (0.25% hydrocortisone, 0.75% fluocortin butyl ester) and non-steroidal (5% bufexamac) dermatologic agents maintenance therapy of eczematous diseases. Zeitschrift für Hautkrankheit 60(3):270–277

Aeschbach R, Loliger J, Scott B C, Murcia A, Butler J, Halliwell B, Arouma O I 1994 Antioxidant actions of thymol, carvacrol, 6-gingerol, zingerone and hydroxytyrosol. Food and Chemical Toxicology 32(1):31–36

Agarwal I, Kharwal H B, Methela C S 1980 Chemical study and antimicrobial properties of essential oil of *Cymbopogon citratus* Linn. Bulletin of Medicoethnobotanical Research 1:401–407

Alam K, Agua T, Maven H et al 1994 Preliminary screening of seaweeds, seagrass and lemongrass oil from Papua New Guinea for antimicrobial and antifungal activity. International Journal of Pharmacology 32(4):396–399

Al-Hader A A, Hasan Z A, Aqel M B 1994 Hyperglycaemic and insulin release inhibitory effects of *Rosmarinus officinalis*. Journal of Ethnopharmacology 43:217–221

Almeida R N, Hiruma C A, Barbosa-Filho J M 1996 Analgesic effect of rotundifolone in rodents. Fitoterapia 67(4):334–338

Altman P M 1989 Australian tea tree oil – a natural antiseptic. Australian Journal of Biotechnology 3(4):247–248

Al-Zuhair H, El-Sayeh B, Ameen H A, Al-Shoora H 1996 Pharmacological studies of cardamom oil in animals. Pharmacological Research 34(1/2):79–82

Anthony 1987 Metabolism of estragole in rat and mouse and influence of dose size on excretion of the proximate carcinogen 1-hydroxy-estragole. Food and Chemical Toxicology 25:799–806 cited by Tisserand R and Balacs T 1995 *Essential Oil Safety: A Guide for Health care Professionals* Churchill Livingstone London pp120

Appleton S M 1997 'Handle with care': an investigation into handling received by preterm infants in intensive care. Journal of Neonatal Nursing 3(3):23–27

Aqel M B 1991 Relaxant effect of the volatile oil of *Rosmarinus officinalis* on tracheal smooth muscle. Journal of Ethnopharmacology 33(1–2):57–62

Aqua Oleum 1993 The essential oil catalogue. Aqua Oleum, Stroud

Arcier M 1992 Aromatherapy. Hamlyn, London

Ariyoshi T, Arakaki M, Ideguchi K, Ishizuka Y, Noda K, Ide H 1975 Studies on the metabolism of *d*-limonene. III Effects of *d*-limonene on the lipids and drug-metabolising enzymes in rats. Xenobiotica 5(1):33–38

Arkko P J, Pakarinen A J, Kari-Koskinen O 1983 Effects of whole body massage on serum protein, electrolyte and hormone concentrations, enzyme activities and haematological parameters. International Journal of Sports Medicine 4:265–267

Aruna K, Sivaramakrishnan V M 1996 Anticarcinogenic effects of the essential oils from cumin, poppy and basil. Phytotherapy Research 10(7):577–580

Asjes E 1993 Managing epilepsy. International Journal of Aromatherapy 5(3):16–19

Assaf M H, Ali A A, Makboul M A et al 1987 Preliminary study of phenolic glycosides from *Origanum marjorana*: quantitative estimation of arbutin: cytotoxic activity of hydroquinone. Planta Medica 53(4):343–345

Atanassova-Shopova S, Roussinov K S 1970 On certain central neurotropic effects of lavender essential oil. Bulletin of the Institute of Physiology 13:69–77

Audicana M, Bernaola G 1994 Occupational contact dermatitis from citrus fruits: lemon essential oils. Contact Dermatitis 31:183–185

Avery M D, Van Arsdale L 1987 Perineal massage: effect on the incidence of episiotomy and laceration in a nulliparous population. Journal of Nurse-Midwifery 32(3):181–184

Aydin S, Ozturk Y, Beis R, Baser K H C 1996 Investigation of *Origanum onites*, *Sideritis congesta* and *Satureja cuneifolila* essential oils for analgesic activity. Phytotherapy Research 10:342–344

Badei A Z M 1992 Antimycotic effect of cardamom essential oil against mycotoxigenic moulds in relation to its chemical composition. Chemie Mikrobiologie Technologie der Lebensmittel 14:177–182

Badia P, Wesensten N, Lammers W et al 1990 Responsiveness to olfactory stimulation presented in sleep. Physiology and Behavior 48(1):87–90

Baker S 1997 Formation and development of the Aromatherapy Organisations Council. Complementary Therapies in Nursing and Midwifery 3:77–80

Bakerink J A, Gospe S M, Dimand R J, Eldridge M W 1996 Multiple organ failure after ingestion of pennyroyal oil from herbal tea in two infants. Pediatrics 98(5):944–947

Balacs T 1991a Essential issues. International Journal of Aromatherapy 3(4):23–25

Balacs T 1991b Research reports. International Journal of Aromatherapy 3(4):29–31

Balacs T 1992a Safety in pregnancy. International Journal of Aromatherapy 4(1):12–15

Balacs T 1992b Dermal crossing. International Journal of Aromatherapy 4(2):23–25

Balacs T 1992c Well oiled pathways. International Journal of Aromatherapy 4(3):14–16

Balacs T 1993 Research reports. International Journal of Aromatherapy 5(3):34

Bannerjee S, Sharma R, Kale R K, Rao A R 1994 Influence of certain essential oils on carcinogen-metabolising enzymes and acid-soluble sulphydryls in mouse liver. Nutrition and Cancer 21(3):263–269

Barr J S, Taslitz N 1970 The influence of back massage on autonomic functions. Physical Therapy 50(12):1679–1691

Barsoum G, Perry E P, Fraser I A 1990 Postoperative nausea is relieved by acupressure. Journal of the Royal Society of Medicine 83:86–89

Bassett I B, Pannowitz D L, Barnetson R S C 1990 A comparative study of tea tree oil versus benzoyl peroxide in the treatment of acne. Medical Journal of Australia 153(8):455–458

Bauer W C, Dracup K A 1987 Physiological effects of back massage in patients with acute myocardial infarction. Focus on Critical Care 14(6):42–46

Beal M W 1992 Acupuncture and related treatment modalities. Part 2: Applications to antepartal and intrapartal care. Journal of Nurse-Midwifery 37(4):260–268

Beccara M A D 1995 Melaleuca oil poisoning in a 17 month old. Veterinary and Human Toxicology 37(6):557–558

Belaiche P 1985a Treatment of vaginal infections of *Candida albicans* with the essential oil of *Melaleuca alternifolia* (Cheel). Phytotherapy 15:13–15

Belaiche P 1985b Treatment of skin infections with the essential oil of *Melaleuca alternifolia* (Cheel). Phytotherapy 15:15–17

Belluomini J, Litt R C, Lee K A et al 1994 Acupressure for nausea and vomiting of pregnancy: a randomized, blinded study. Obstetrics and Gynecology 84(2):245–248

Belman S 1983 Onion and garlic oils inhibit tumor promotion. Carcinogenesis 4(8):1063–1065

Bennett A, Stamford I F, Tavares I A et al 1988 The biological activity of eugenol, a major constituent of nutmeg (*Myristica fragrans*): studies on prostaglandins, the intestine and other tissues. Phytotherapy Research 2(3):124–130

Bensoussan A 1991 The vital meridian. Churchill Livingstone, London

Betts T 1994 Sniffing the breeze. Aromatherapy Quarterly 40:19–23

Bhatnagae M, Kapur K K, Jalees S, Sharma S K 1993 Laboratory evaluation of insecticidal properties of *Ocimum basilicum* Linnaeus and *Ocimum sanctum* Linnaeus plant's essential oils and their major constituents against vector mosquito species. Journal of Entomological Research 17(1):21–26

Bilsland D, Strong A 1990 Allergic contact dermatitis from the essential oil of French marigold (*Tagetes patula*) in an aromatherapist. Contact Dermatitis 23:55–56

Birch E R 1986 The experience of touch received during labour: postpartum perceptions of therapeutic value. Journal of Nurse-Midwifery 31(6):270–276

Boatto G, Pintore G, Palomba M 1994 Composition and antibacterial activity of *Inula helenium* and *Rosmarinus officinalis* essential oils. Fitoterapia 65(3):279–280

Bourhis B, Soenen A-M 1973 Recherches sur l'action psychotropes de quelques substances aromatiques utilisées en alimentation. Food and Cosmetics Toxicology 11:1–9

Bowers-Clarke M 1993 Baby massage. New Generation 12(3):4–5

Boyd E M, Sheppard E P 1968 The effect of steam inhalation of volatile oils on the output and composition of respiratory tract fluid. Journal of Pharmacology and Experimental Therapeutics 163(1):250–256

Boyd E M, Sheppard P 1970 Nutmeg oil and camphene as inhaled expectorants. Archives of Otolaryngology 92(4):372–378

Boyland E, Chasseau F 1970 The effects of some carbonyl compounds on rat liver glutathione levels. Biochemical Pharmacology 19:1526–1528

Brandao F M 1986 Occupational allergy to lavender oil. Contact Dermatitis 15(4):249–250

British Medical Association 1993 Complementary medicine: new approaches to good practice. Oxford University Press, Oxford

Brud W, Konopacka-Brud I 1994 Rose oils. International Journal of Aromatherapy 6(2):12–16

Buchbauer G, Jirovetz L, Jager W et al 1991 Aromatherapy: evidence for sedative effects of the essential oil of lavender after inhalation. Zeitshrift für Naturforschung C 46(11–12):1067–1072

Buchbauer G, Jirovetz L, Jager W et al 1993 Fragrance compounds and essential oils with sedative effects upon inhalation. Journal of Pharmaceutical Sciences 82(6):660–664

Buckle J 1993 Aromatherapy. Does it matter which lavender essential oil is used? Nursing Times 89(20):32–35

Budd S 1992 Traditional Chinese medicine in obstetrics. Midwives Chronicle 105(1253):140–143

Burns E, Blamey C 1994 Using aromatherapy in childbirth. Nursing Times 90(9):54–60

Cabo J, Crespo M E, Jimenez J, Zarzuelo A 1986 The spasmolytic activity of various aromatic plants from the province of Granada. The activity of the major components of their essential oils. Plantes Médicinales et Phytotherapie 20(3):213–218

Calnan C D 1976 Cinnamon dermatitis from an ointment. Contact Dermatitis 2:167–170

Cardullo A C, Ruszkowski A M, Deleto V A 1989 Allergic contact dermatitis resulting from sensitivity to citrus peel, geraniol and citral. Journal of the American Academy of Dermatology 21(2):395–397

Carle R, Gomaa K 1992 The medicinal use of *Matricariae flos*. British Journal of Phytotherapy 2(4):147–153

Carola R, Harley J P, Noback C R 1992 Human anatomy and physiology, 2nd edn. McGraw Hill, New York

Carson C F, Riley T V 1994 Susceptibility of *Propionibacterium* acnes to the essential oil of *Melaleuca alternifolia*. Letters in Applied Microbiology 19(1):24–25

Carson C F, Riley T V 1995 Antimicrobial activity of the major components of the essential oil of *Melaleuca alternifolia*. Journal of Applied Bacteriology 78(3):264–269

Carson C F, Cookson B D, Farrelly H D, Riley T V 1995 Susceptibility of methicillin-resistant *Staphylococcus aureus* to the essential oil of *Melaleuca alternifolia*. Journal of Antimicrobial Chemotherapy 35(3):421–424

Carson C F, Hammer K A, Riley T V 1996 In vitro activity of the essential oil of *Melaleuca alternifolia* against *Streptococcus* spp. Journal of Antimicrobial Chemotherapy 37(6):1177–1181

Chadha A, Madyastha K M 1984 Metabolism of geraniol and linalool in the rat and effects on liver and lung microsomal enzymes. Xenobiotica 14:365–374

Chaplin J 1996 The benefits of baby massage. Community Health Action 39:9–11

Chokechaijaroenporn O, Bunyapraphatsara N, Kongchuensin S 1994 Mosquito repellent activities of *Ocimum* volatile oils. Phytomedicine 1:135–139

Coelho-de-Souza A N, Barata E L, Magalhaes P J C, Lima C C, Leal-Cardaso J H 1997 Effects of the essential oil of *Croton zehntneri* and its constituent estragole on intestinal smooth muscle. Phytotherapy Research 11:299–304

Cooke A, Cooke M D 1991 An investigation into the antimicrobial properties of manuka and kanuka oil. Cawthron Institute Report, February

Cooperative Group for the Essential Oil of Garlic 1986 The effect of the essential oil of garlic on hyperlipaemia and platelet aggregation – an analysis of 308 cases. Journal of Traditional Chinese Medicine 6(2):117–120

Cornwell P A, Barry B W 1994 Sesquiterpene components of volatile oils as skin penetration enhancers for the hydrophililc permeant 5-fluorouracil. Journal of Pharmacy and Pharmacology 46(4):261–269

Craig J O 1953 Poisoning by the volatile oils in childhood. Archives of Disease in Childhood 28:259–267

Cruz T, Jimenez J, Zarzuelo A, Cabo M M 1989 The spasmolytic activity of the essential oil of *Thymus baeticus* in rats. Phytotherapy Research 3(3):106–108

Cullen S I, Tonkin A, May F E 1974 Allergic contact dermatitis to compound tincture of benzoin spray. Journal of Trauma 14(4):348–350

Curran F 1996 Massage, a skill at our fingertips. Modern Midwife 6(7):11

Dale A, Cornwell S 1994 The role of lavender oil in relieving perineal discomfort following childbirth: a blind randomized clinical trial. Journal of Advanced Nursing 19(1):89–96

Davis P 1988 Aromatherapy – an A–Z. C W Daniel, Saffron Walden

Day J A, Mason R R, Chesrow S E 1987 Effect of massage on serum level of beta-endorphins and beta-lipotropin in healthy adults. Physical Therapy 67(6):926–930

De Aloysio D, Penacchioni P 1992 Morning sickness control in early pregnancy by Neiguan point acupressure. Obstetrics and Gynecology 80(5):852–854

Deans S G, Ritchie G 1987 Antibacterial properties of plant essential oils. International Journal of Food Microbiology 5:165–180

Deans S G, Svoboda K P 1990 The antimicrobial properties of marjoram (*Origanum marjorana* L.) volatile oil. Flavour and Fragrance Journal 5(3):187–190

Deans S G, Noble R C, Penzes L, Imre S G 1993 Promotional effects of plant volatile oils on the polyunsaturated fatty acid status during ageing. Age 16:71–74

De Groot A C 1996 Airborne allergic contact dermatitis from tea tree oil. Contact Dermatitis 35(5):304–305

De Groot A C, Weyland J W 1992 Systemic contact dermatitis from tea tree oil. Contact Dermatitis 27(4):279–280

De Groot A C, Weyland J W 1993 Contact allergy to tea tree oil. Contact Dermatitis 28(2):309

de la Puerta R, Herrera M D 1995 Spasmolytic action of the essential oil of *Achillea ageratum* L. in rats. Phytotherapy Research 9(2):150–152 de la Puerta R, Saenz M T, Garcia M D 1993 Choleretic effect of the essential oil from *Helichrysum picardii* Boiss. and reuter in rats. Phytotherapy Research 7:376–377

Delgado I F, Carvalho S H P, Nogueira A C M et al 1993a Study on the embryo-fetotoxicity of beta-myrcene in the rat. Food and Chemical Toxicology 31(1):31–35

Delgado I F, De Almeida Nogueira C M, Souza C A M, Costa A M N, Figueiredo L H 1993b Peri- and post-natal developmental toxicity of beta-myrcene in the rat. Food and Chemical Toxicology 31(9):623–628

Demetriou A A, Seifter E, Levenson S M 1974 Effect of vitamin A and citral on peritoneal adhesion formation. Journal of Surgical Research 17:325–329

Department of Genito-urinary Medicine 1991 Tea tree oil and anaerobic (bacterial) vaginosis. The Lancet 337(8736):300

Department of Health 1993 Changing childbirth: Report of the expert maternity group. HMSO, London

de Roiste A, Bushnell I W R 1995 The immediate gastric effects of a tactile stimulation programme on premature infants. Journal of Reproductive and Infant Psychology 13(1):57–62

de Roiste A, Bushnell I, Burns J 1995 TAC-TIC: how do special care baby unit babies react to it? British Journal of Midwifery 3(1):8–10, 12–15

Dew M J, Evans B K, Rhodes J 1984 Peppermint oil for irritable bowel syndrome: a multicentre trial. British Journal of Clinical Practice 38(11–12):394, 398

Domokos J D, Hethelyi E, Palinkas J, Szirmal S 1997 Essential oil of rosemary (*Rosmarinus officinalis*) of Hungarian origin. Journal of Essential Oil Research 9:41–45

Dooms-Goossens A, Degreef H, Holvoet C, Maertens M 1977 Turpentine-induced hypersensitivity to peppermint oil. Contact Dermatitis 3(6):304–308

Dube S, Upadhyay P D, Tripathi S C 1989 Antifungal, physiochemical and insect-repelling activity of essential oil of *Ocimum basilicum*. Canadian Journal of Botany 67(7):2085–2087

Dundee J W, Yang J 1990 Prolongation of the antiemetic action of P6 acupuncture by acupressure in patients having cancer chemotherapy. Journal of the Royal Society of Medicine 83:360–362

Dundee J W, Sourial F B R, Ghaly R G 1988 P6 acupuncture reduces morning sickness. Journal of the Royal Society of Medicine 81(8):456–457

Dunn C, Sleep J, Collett D 1995 Sensing an improvement: an experimental study to evaluate the use of aromatherapy, massage and rest in an intensive care unit. Journal of Advanced Nursing 21(1):34–40

Duthie H L 1981 The effect of peppermint oil on colonic activity in man. British Journal of Surgery 68:820

Elisabetsky E, Marschner J, Souza D O 1995 Effects of linalool on glutamatergic system in the rat cerebral cortex. Neurochemical Research 20(4):461–465

Elisha N et al 1988 Effects of *Jasminum officinale* flowers on the central nervous system of the mouse. International Journal of Crude Drug Research 26(4):221–227

Elson C E, Maltzman T H, Boston J L, Tanner M A, Gould M N 1988 Anticarcinogenic activity of *d*-limonene during the initiation and promotion/progression stages of DMBA-induced rat mammary carcinogenesis. Carcinogenesis 9(2):331–332

Elson C E, Underbakke G L, Hanson P et al 1989 Impact of lemongrass oil, an essential oil, on serum cholesterol. Lipids 24(8):677–679

El Tahir K E H, Ashour M M S, Al-Harbi M M 1993a The cardiovascular actions of the volatile oil of the black seed (*Nigella sativa*) in rats: elucidation of the mechanism of action. General Pharmacology 24(5):1123–1131

El Tahir K E H, Ashour M M S, Al-Harbi M M 1993b The respiratory effects of the volatile oil of the black seed (*Nigella sativa*) in guinea pigs: elucidation of the mechanism(s) of action. General Pharmacology 24(5):1115–1122

Eriksson K, Levin J 1990 Identification of *cis*- and *trans*-verbenol in human urine after occupational exposure to terpenes. International Archives of Occupational and Environmental Health 62:379–383

Ernst E, Matrai A, Magyarosy L et al 1987 Massage causes changes in blood fluidity. Physiotherapy 73(1):43–45

Evans A T, Samuels S N, Marshall C et al 1993 Suppression of pregnancy-induced nausea and vomiting with sensory afferent stimulation. Journal of Reproductive Medicine 38(8):603–606

Falk-Filipsson A 1993 *d*-Limonene exposure to humans by inhalation: uptake, distribution, elimination and effects on the pulmonary system. Journal of Toxicology and Environmental Health 38:77–88

Fang H J, Su X L, Liu X Y et al 1989 Studies on the chemical components and anti-tumour action of the volatile oils from *Pelargonium graveolens*. Yao Hsueh Hsueh Pao 24(5):366–371

Farag R S, Daw Z Y, Hewedi F M, El-Baroty G S A 1989 Antimicrobial activity of some Egyptian spice essential oils. Journal of Food Protection 52(9):665–667

Farrell M 1994 Jottings from journals. Aromatherapy World, Summer 1994:26

Farrow J 1990 Massage therapy and nursing care. Nursing Standard 4(17):26–28

Feinblatt H M 1960 Cajeput-type oil for the treatment of furunculosis. Journal of the National Medical Association 1:32–34

Ferley J P, Poutignat N, Zmirou D, Azzopardi Y, Balducci F 1989 Prophylactic aromatherapy for supervening infections in patients with chronic bronchitis. Statistical evaluation conducted in clinics against a placebo. Phytotherapy Research 3(3):97–100

Ferrell-Torry A T, Glick O J 1993 The use of therapeutic massage as a nursing intervention to modify anxiety and the perception of cancer pain. Cancer Nursing 16(2):93–101

Field T M, Schanburg S M, Scadafi F et al 1986 Tactile/kinesthetic stimulation effects on preterm neonates. Pediatrics 77(5):654–658

Field T, Morrow C, Vaideon C et al 1993 Massage reduces anxiety in child and adolescent psychiatric patients. International Journal of Alternative and Complementary Medicine 11(7):22–27

Foundation for Integrated Medicine 1997 Integrated healthcare: a way forward for the next five years? Foundation for Integrated Medicine, London

Fowler P, Wall M 1997 COSHH and CHIPS: ensuring the safety of aromatherapy. Complementary Therapies in Medicine 2(5):112–115

Fowler P, Wall M 1998 Aromatherapy, control of substances hazardous to health (COSHH) and assessment of chemical risk. Complementary Therapies in Medicine 3(3):85–93

Fraser J, Kerr J R 1993 Psychophysiological effects of back massage on elderly institutionalised patients. Journal of Advanced Nursing 18:238–245

Gabbrielli G, Loggini F, Cioni P L et al 1988 Activity of lavandin essential oil against non-tubercular opportunistic rapid growth mycobacteria. Pharmacological Research Communications, December (supplement 5):37–40

Galal E E, Adel M S, El-Sherif S, Girgis A N, Bofael N 1973 Evaluation of certain volatile oils for their antifungal properties. Journal of Drug Research 5(2):235–245

Gamez M J, Jimenez J, Navarro C, Zarzuelo A 1990 Study of the essential oil of *Lavandula dentata*. Pharmazie 45:69

Garg S C, Dengre S L 1986 Antibacterial activity of essential oil of *Tagetes erecta* Linn. Hindustan Antibiotics Bulletin 28(1–4):27–29

Garland D 2000 The uses of hydrotherapy in today's midwifery practice. In: Tiran D, Mack S (eds) Complementary therapies for pregnancy and childbirth, 2nd edn. Baillière Tindall, London, pp 225–237

Giachetti D, Taddei E, Taddei I 1988 Pharmacological activity of essential oils on Oddi's sphincter. Planta Medica 54(5):389–392

Ginsberg F, Famaey J P 1987 A double-blind study of topical massage with Rado-salil ointment in mechanical low-back pain. Journal of International Medical Research 15:148–153

Glowania H J, Raulin C, Soboda M 1987 Effect of chamomile on wound healing – a clinical double-blind study. Zeitschrift für Hautkrankheit 62(17):1267–1271

Gobel H, Schmidt G, Soyka D 1994 Effect of peppermint and eucalyptus oil preparations on neurophysiological and experimental algesimetric headache parameters. Cephalalgia 14:228–234

Gobel H, Schmidt G, Dworschak M, Stolze H, Heuss D 1995 Essential plant oils and headache mechanisms. Phytomedicine 2(2):93–102

Goldberg J, Sullivan S J, Seaborne D E 1992 The effect of two intensities of massage on H-reflex amplitude. Physical Therapy 72(6):449–457

Guerra P, Aguilar A, Urbina F et al 1987 Contact dermatitis to geraniol in a leg ulcer. Contact Dermatitis 16(5):298–299

Guillemain J, Rousseau A, Delaveau P 1989 Neurodepressive effects of the essential oil of *Lavandula angustifolia* Mill. Annales Pharmaceutiques Françaises 47(6):337–343

Gui-Yuan Y, Wei W 1994 Clinical studies on treatment of coronary heart disease with *Valeriana officinalis* var. latifolia. Chung Ku C H I C H Tsa Chih 14(9):540–542 (cited in Harris B 1997 Aromatherapy database. Essential Oil Resource Consultants, St Germain le Guillaume, France)

Gundidza M, Chinyanganya F, Mavi S 1993 Antimicrobial activity of the essential oil from *Eucalyptus maidenii*. Planta Medica 59 (supplement):A705

Gurr F W, Scroggie J G 1965 Eucalyptus oil poisoning treated by dialysis and mannitol infusion, with an appendix on the analysis of biological fluids for alcohol and eucalyptol. Australasian Annals of Medicine 14(3):238–249

Hajji F, Fkih-Tetouani S 1993 Antimicrobial activity of twenty one eucalyptus essential oils. Fitoterapia 64(1):71–77

Hammer K A, Carson C F, Riley T V 1996 Susceptibility of transient and commensal skin flora to the essential oil of *Melaleuca alternifolia* (tea tree oil). Australian Journal of Infection Control 24(3):186–189

Hardcastle A B, Hardcastle P T, Taylor C J 1996 Influence of peppermint oil on absorptive and secretory processes in rat small intestine. Gut 39:214–219

Hardy M 1991 Sweet scented dreams. International Journal of Aromatherapy 3(2):12–13

Harrison L L, Leeper J D, Yoon M 1990 Effects of early parent touch on preterm infants' heart rates and arterial oxygen saturation levels. Journal of Advanced Nursing 15(8):877–885

Hartnoll G, Moore D, Douek D 1993 Near fatal ingestion of oil of cloves. Archives of Disease in Childhood 69:392–393

Hedstrom L W, Newton N 1986 Touch in labour: a comparison of cultures and eras. Birth 13(3):181–186

Helders P J M, Cats B P, van der Net J et al 1988 The effects of a tactile stimulation/range-finding programme on the development of very low birth weight infants during initial hospitalization. Child: Care, Health and Development 14(5):341–353

Henry J, Rusius C W, Davies M, Veazey-French T 1994 Lavender for night sedation of people with dementia. International Journal of Aromatherapy 6(2):28–30

Hethelyi E, Kaposi P, Domonkos J, Kernoczi Z 1987 GC/MS investigation of the essential oil of *Rosmarinus officinalis* L. Acta Pharmaceutica Hungarica 57(3–4):159–169

Hill C F 1993 Is massage beneficial to critically ill patients in intensive care? A critical review. Journal of Intensive Critical Care Nursing. 9:116–121

Hills J M, Aaronson P I 1991 The mechanism of action of peppermint oil on gastrointestinal muscle. An analysis using patch clamp electrophysiology and isolated tissue pharmacology in rabbit and guinea pig. Gastroenterology 10(1):55–65

Hiroi T, Miyazaki Y, Kobayashi Y, Imaoka S, Funae Y 1995 Induction of hepatic P-450s in rat by essential wood and leaf oils. Xenobiotica 25(5):457–467

Hmamouch M, Tantaoui-Elaraki A, Es-Safu N, Agoumi A 1990 Illustration of antibacterial and antifungal properties of Eucalyptus essential oils. Plantes Médicinales et Phytothérapie 24(4):278–289

Hof S, Ammon T 1989 Negative inotropic action of rosemary oil, 1,8-cineole and bornyl acetate. Planta Medica 55(1):106–107

Holmes P 1994 Rose – the water goddess. International Journal of Aromatherapy 6(2):8–11

Holmes P 1998 Jasmine. The queen of the night. International Journal of Aromatherapy 8(4):8–12

Hovind H, Nielson S L 1974 Effect of massage on blood flow in skeletal muscle. Scandinavian Journal of Rehabilitation Medicine 6:74–77

Hudson R 1996 The value of lavender for rest and sleep in the elderly. Complementary Therapies in Medicine 4:52–57

Hyde E 1989 Acupressure therapy for morning sickness. A controlled clinical trial. Journal of Nurse-Midwifery 34(4):171–178

Imberger I, Rupp J, Karamat C, Buchbauer G 1993 Effects of essential oils on human attentional processes. Programme abstracts – 24th International Symposium on Essential Oils

Ineson M 1995 The psychological and physiological effects of massage on full term, 'normal' babies and their participating parents. Journal of the Association of Chartered Physiotherapists in Women's Health 77 (August): 3–7

International School of Aromatherapy 1993 A safety guide on the use of essential oils. Natural by Nature, London

Isaac O 1979 Pharmacological investigations with compounds of chamomile. On the pharmacology of alpha–bisabolol and bisabolol oxides (review). Planta Medica 35:118–124

Isherwood D 1994 Baby massage groups. New Generation 12(3):4–6

Jacobs M R, Hornfeldt C S 1994 Melaleuca oil poisoning. Clinical Toxicology 32(4):461–464

Jager W, Buchbauer G, Jirovetz L 1992 Evidence of the sedative effects of neroli oil, citronellal and phenylethyl acetate on mice. Journal of Essential Oil Research 4:387–394

Jakovlev V, Flaskamp I, Flaskamp E 1983 Pharmacological investigations with compounds of chamomile VI. Investigations on the antiphlogistic effects of chamazulene and matricine. Planta Medica 49:67–73

Jalsenjak V, Peljnjak S, Kusttrak D 1987 Microcapsules of sage oil: essential oil content and antimicrobial activity. Pharmazie 42(6):419–420

James W D, White S W, Yanklowitz B 1984 Allergic contact dermatitis to compound tincture of benzoin. Journal of the American Academy of Dermatology 5(1):847–850

Janssens J, Laekeman G M, Pieters L A et al 1990 Nutmeg oil: identification and quantitation of its most active constituents as inhibitors of platelet aggregation. Journal of Ethnopharmacology 29(2):179–188

Jenson O K, Nielson F F, Vosmar L 1990 An open study comparing manual therapy with the use of cold packs in the treatment of post-traumatic headache. Cephalagia 10:241–249

Jirovetz L, Buchbauer G, Jager W et al 1992 Analysis of fragrance compounds in blood samples of mice by gas chromatography, mass spectrometry, GC/FTIR and GC/AES after inhalation of sandalwood oil. Biomedical Chromatography 6(3):133–134

Johanson R B, Spencer S A, Rolfe P et al 1992 Effect of post-delivery care on neonatal body temperature. Acta Paediatrica 81(11):859–863

Johnson E 2000 Shiatsu. In: Tiran D, Mack S (eds) Complementary therapies for pregnancy and childbirth, 2nd edn. Baillière Tindall, London, pp 189–213

Jori A, Bianchietti A, Prestini P E 1969 Effects of essential oils on drug metabolism. Biochemical Pharmacology 18(9):2081–2085

Joshi D J, Dikshit R K, Mansuri S M 1987 Gastrointestinal actions of garlic oil. Phytotherapy Research 1(3):140–141

Juven B J, Kanner J, Schved F, Weisslowicz H 1994 Factors that interact with the antibacterial action of thyme essential oil and its active constituents. Journal of Applied Bacteriology 76:626–631

Kaada B, Torsteinbo O 1989 Increase of plasma beta-endorphins in connective tissue massage. General Pharmacology 20(4):487–489

Kallan C 1991 Probing the power of common scents. Prevention 43(10):38

Karamat E, Imberger J, Buchbauer G et al 1992 Excitory and sedative effects of essential oils on human reaction time performance. Chemical Senses 17(4):847

Kikuchi A, Tsuchiya T, Tanida M et al 1989 Stimulant-like ingredients in absolute jasmine. Chemical Senses 14(2): 304

Kikuchi A, Tanida M, Uenoyama S, Abe T, Yamaguchi H 1991 Effect of odors on cardiac response patterns in a reaction time task. Chemical Senses 16:183

Kilibarda V, Nanusevic N, Dogovic N, Ivanic R, Savin K 1996 Content of the essential oil of the carrot and its antibacterial activity. Pharmazie 51:777–778

Kirov M, Burkova T, Kapurdov V, Spasovski M 1988a Rose oil. Lipotropic effect in modelled fatty dystrophy of the liver. (Morphological and enzymohistochemical study.) Medico Biologica Information 3:18–22

Kirov M, Bainova A, Spasovski M 1988b Rose oil. Acute and subacute oral toxicity Medico Biologica Information 3:8–14

Knasko S C 1992 Ambient odor's effect on creativity, mood and perceived health. Chemical Senses 17(1):27–35

Knight T E, Hausen B M 1994 Melaleuca oil (tea tree) dermatitis. Journal of the American Academy of Dermatology 30(3):423–427

Kobal G et al 1992 Differences in human chemosensory evoked potentials to olfactory and somatosensory chemical stimuli presented to left and right nostrils. Chemical Senses 17(3):233–244

Kovar K A, Gropper B, Friess D Svendsen A 1987 Blood levels of 1,8-cineole and locomotor activity of mice after inhalation and oral administration of rosemary oil. Planta Medica 53(4):315–318

Kubler S, Wabner D 1994 A museum for the rose. Aromatherapy Quarterly 41:21–25

Kuhn C M, Schanberg S M, Field T et al 1991 Tactile–kinesthetic stimulation effects on sympathetic and adrenocortical function in preterm infants. Journal of Pediatrics 119(3):434–440

Kumar A, Sharma V D, Sing A K, Singh K 1988 Antibacterial properties of different Eucalyptus oils. Fitoterapia 59(2):141–144

Labrecque M, Marcoux S, Pinault J J et al 1994 Prevention of perineal trauma by perineal massage during pregnancy: a pilot study. Birth 21(1):20–25

Lam L K, Zheng B 1991 Effects of essential oils on glutathione-S-transferase activity in mice. Journal of Agricultural and Food Chemistry 39:660–662

Larrondo J V, Calvo M A 1991 Effect of essential oils on Candida albicans: a scanning electron microscope study. Biomedical Letters 46(184):269–272

Lavabre M 1990 Aromatherapy workbook. Healing Arts Press, Rochester, USA

Lawless J 1992 The encyclopaedia of essential oils. Element Books, Shaftesbury

Lawless J 1994 Scent, soul and psyche. Aromatherapy Quarterly 42:17–21

Leicester R J, Hunt R H 1982 Peppermint oil to reduce colonic spasm during endoscopy. Lancet 2(8305):989

Le May A 1986 The human connection. Nursing Times 19 November 1986:28–30

Lesesne C B 1992 The postoperative use of wound adhesives. Gum mastic *versus* benzoin, USP. Journal of Dermatologic Surgery and Oncology 18(11):990

Leung A Y 1980 Encyclopaedia of common natural ingredients used in food, drugs and cosmetics. John Wiley, New York

Lichy R, Herzberg E 1993 The waterbirth handbook. Gateway Books, Bath

Lim P 1996 Baby massage. British Journal of Midwifery 4(8):439–441

Lis-Balchin M, Hart S, Deans S G, Eaglesham E 1995 Potential agrochemical and medicinal usage of essential oils of *Pelargonium* species. Journal of Herbs, Spices and Medicinal Plants 3(2):11–22

Lis-Balchin M, Deans S G, Hart S 1996a Bioactivity of New Zealand medicinal plant essential oils. Acta Horticulturae 426:13–29

Lis-Balchin M, Hart S, Deans S G, Eaglesham E 1996b Comparison of the pharmacological and antimicrobial action of commercial plant essential oils. Journal of Herbs, Spices and Medical Plants 4(2):69–86

Lis-Balchin M, Deans S G, Hart S L 1996c Bioactivity of geranium oils from different commercial sources. Journal of Essential Oil Research 8:281–290

Lorenzetti B B, Souza G E, Sarti S J et al 1991 Myrcene mimics the peripheral analgesic activity of lemongrass tea. Journal of Ethnopharmacology 34(1):43–48

Lorig T S, Roberts M 1990 Odor and cognitive alteration of the contingent negative variation. Chemical Senses 15:537–545

Lorig T S et al 1993 Visual event-related potentials during odour labelling. Chemical Senses 18(4):379–387

Low D, Rawal B D, Griffin W J 1974 Antibacterial action of the essential oils of some Australian Myrtaceae with special references to the activity of chromatographic fractions of oil of *Eucalyptus citriodora*. Planta Medica 26:184–189

Ludvigson H W, Rottman T R 1989 Effect of ambient odors of lavender and cloves on cognition, memory, affect and mood. Chemical Senses 14(4):525–536

Lyrenas S, Lutsch H, Hetta J et al 1987 Acupuncture before delivery: effect on labor. Gynecologic and Obstetric Investigation 24(4):217–224

Madyastha K M, Srivatsan V 1987 Metabolism of beta-myrcene in vivo and in vitro: its effects on rat liver microsomal enzymes. Xenobiotica 17(5):539–549

Mason M 1996 Baby massage: the importance of touch. Johnson & Johnson, Maidenhead, Berks

Manley C H 1993 Psychophysiological effect of odour. Critical Reviews in Food Science and Nutrition 33(1):57–62

Mann R J 1982 Benzoin sensitivity. Contact Dermatitis 8(4):263

Marsden K 1991 The aromatherapy phenomenon. International Journal of Aromatherapy 3(4):6–9

McArdle M 1992 Rosewood in pre-eclampsia. International Journal of Aromatherapy 4(1):33 (letter)

McGeorge B C, Steele M C 1991 Allergic contact dermatitis of the nipple from Roman chamomile ointment. Contact Dermatitis 24(2):139–140

McKechnie A A, Wilson F, Watson N, Scott D 1983 Anxiety states: a preliminary report on the value of connective tissue massage. Journal of Psychosomatic Research 27(2):125–129

Meeker H G, Linke H A 1988 The antibacterial action of eugenol, thyme oil and related essential oils used in dentistry. Compendium 9(1):34–35, 38

Mehrotra S, Rawat A K S, Shome U 1993 Antimicrobial activity of the essential oils of some Indian *Artemesia* species. Fitoterapia 64(1):65–68

Melegari M, Albasini A, Pecorari G, Vampa G, Rinaldi M 1989 Chemical characteristics a nd pharmacological properties of the essential oil of *Anthemis nobilis*. Fitoterapia 59(6):449–455

Melzig M, Teuscher E 1991 Investigations of the influence of essential oils and their main components on the adenosine uptake by cultivated endothelial cells. Planta Medica 57(1):41–42

Menella J A, Johnson A, Beauchamp G K 1995 Garlic ingestion by pregnant women alters the odor of amniotic fluid. Chemical Senses 20(2):207–209

Meyer J 1970 Accidents due to tanning cosmetics with a base of bergamot oil. Bulletin de la Societe Francaise de Dermatologie et de Syphiligraphie 77(6):881–884

Miller T M, Wittstock U, Lindequist U, Teuscher E 1996 Effects of some components of the essential oil of chamomile, *Chamomilla recutita*, on histamine release from rat mast cells. Planta Medica 62(1):60–61

Millet Y, Jouglard J, Steinmetz M D, Tognetti P, Joanny P, Arditti J 1981 Toxicity of some essential plant oils. Clinical and experimental study. Clinical Toxicology 18(12):1485–1498

Minchin M 1994 Geranium. When there were no more cabbage leaves. Australian Lactation Consultants Association (ALCA) News 5(1):8–10

Mishra P, Chauhan C S 1984 Antimicrobial studies of the essential oil of the berries of *Juniperus macropoda* Boiss. Hindustan Antibiotics Bulletin 26(1):38–40

Misra N, Batra S, Mishra D 1988 Fungitoxic properties of the essential oil of *Citrus lemon* (L.) Burm. against a few dermatophytes. Mycoses 31(7):380–382

Miyazaki Y, Takeuchi S, Yatagi M, Kobayashi S 1991 The effect of essential oils on mood in humans. Chemical Senses 16(1):184

Moorthy B 1991 Toxicity and metabolism of *R*-pulegone in rats: its effects on hepatic cytochrome P-450 in vivo and in vitro. Indian Institute of Science 71(1):76–78

Moran A, Martin M L, Montero M J, Ortiz de Urbina A V, Sevilla M A, San Roman L 1989 Analgesic, antipyretic and anti-inflammatory activity of the essential oil of *Artemesia caerulescens* subsp. *gallica*. Journal of Ethnopharmacology 27(3):307–317

Morelli M, Seaborne D E, Sullivan S J 1990 Changes in H-reflex amplitude during massage of triceps surae in healthy subjects. Journal of Orthopaedic and Sports Physical Therapy 12(2):55–59

Mumm A H, Morens D M, Diwan A R 1993 Zoster after shiatsu massage. Lancet 341:447

Mynaugh P A 1991 A randomized study of two methods of teaching perineal massage: effects on practice rates, episiotomy rates and lacerations. Birth 18(3):153–159

Nagai H, Nakagawa M, Nakamura M, Fujii W, Inui T, Asakura Y 1991 Effects of odors on humans. II Reducing effects of mental stress and fatigue. Chemical Senses 16:198

Naganuma M, Hirose S, Nakayama Y et al 1985 A study of the phototoxicity of lemon oil. Archives of Dermatological Research 278(1):31–36

Nakagawa M, Nagai H, Inui T 1992 Evaluation of drowsiness by EEGs – odors controlling drowsiness. Fragrance Journal 20(10):68–72

Nasel C, Nasel B, Samec P et al 1994 Functional imaging of effects of fragrances on the human brain after prolonged inhalation. Chemical Senses 19(4):359–364

Nash P, Gould S R, Bernado D F 1986 Peppermint oil does not relieve the pain of irritable bowel syndrome. British Journal of Clinical Practice 40(7):292–293

Ndounga M, Ouamba J M 1997 Antibacterial and antifungal activities of essential oils of *Ocimum gratissimum* and *O. basilicum*. Fitoterapia 68(2):190–191

NHS Confederation 1997 Complementary medicine in the NHS: managing the issues. NHS Confederation, Birmingham

Nikolaevski V V, Kononova N S, Pertsovskii A I, Shinkarchuk I F 1990 Effect of essential oils on the course of experimental atherosclerosis. Patologicheskaia Fiziologiiai Eksperimentalnaia Terapiia (Moskva) 5:52–53 (cited in Harris B 1997 Aromatherapy database. Essential Oil Resource Consultants, St Germain le Guillaume, France, p 30)

Nissen H P, Biltz H, Kreysel H W 1988 Profilometry, a method for the assessment of the therapeutic effectiveness of Kamillosan ointment. Zeitschrift für Hautkrankheit 63(3):184–190

Nogueira A C, Carvalho R R, Souza C A M, Chahoud I, Paumgartten F J R 1995 Study on the embryofoeto-toxicity of citral in the rat. Toxicology 96(2):105–113

Occhiuto F, Circosta C 1996a Cardiovascular properties of the non-volatile total residue from the essential oil of *Citrus bergamia*. International Journal of Pharmacology 34(2):128–133

Occhiuto F, Circosta C 1996b Antianginal and antiarrhythmic effects of bergamottine, a furocoumarin isolated from bergamot oil. Phytotherapy Research 10(6):491–496

Occhiuto F, Limardi F, Circosta C 1995 Effects of the non-volatile residue from the essential oil of *Citrus bergamia* on the central nervous system. International Journal of Pharmacology 33(3):198–203

Ogunlana E O, Hoglund S, Onawunmi G, Skold O 1987 Effects of lemongrass oil on the morphological characteristics and peptidoglycan synthesis of *Escherichia coli* cells. Microbios 50:43–59

Okugawa H, Ueda R, Matsumoto K, Kawanishi K, Kato A 1995 Effect of alpha-santalol and beta-santalol from sandalwood on the central nervous system in mice Phytomedicine 2(2):119–126

Onawunmi G O 1988 *In vitro* studies on the antibacterial activity of phenoxyethanol in combination with lemongrass oil. Pharmazie 43(1):42–43

Onawunmi G O 1989 Antifungal activity of lemongrass oil. International Journal of Crude Drug Research 27(2):121–126

Onawunmi G O, Ogunlana E O 1986 A study of the antibacterial activity of the essential oil of lemon grass (*Cymbopogon citratus*) (D.C.) Stapf. International Journal of Crude Drug Research 24(2):64–68

Onawunmi G O, Yisak W A, Ogunlana E O 1984 Antibacterial constituents in the essential oil of *Cymbopogon citratus* (D.C.) Stapf. Ethnopharmacology 12(3):279–286

Orafidiya L O 1993 The effect of auto-oxidation of lemongrass oil on its antibacterial activity. Phytotherapy Research 7:269–271

Ozaki Y, Soedigdo S 1988 Cholagogic effect of zingiber plants obtained from Indonesia. Shoyakugaku Zasshi 42(4):333–336 (cited in Harris B 1997 Aromatherapy database. Essential Oil Resource Consultants, St Germain le Guillaume, France, p 112)

Pages N, Fournier G, Chamorro G, Salazar M, Paris M, Boudine C 1989 Teratological evaluation of *Juniperus sabina* essential oil in mice. Planta Medica 55(2):144–146

Pages N, Fournier G, Le Luyer F, Marques M C 1990 Essential oils and their potential teratogenic properties: the case of *Eucalyptus globulus* essential oil – preliminary study on mice. Plantes Médicinales et Phytothérapie 24(1):21–26

Pages N, Fournier G, Baduel C, Tur N, Rusnac M 1996 Sabinyl acetate, the main component of *Juniperus sabina* L'Herit. essential oil, is responsible for anti-implantation effect. Phytotherapy Research 10(7):438–440

Pandit V A, Shelef L A 1994 Sensitivity of *Listeria monocytogenes* to rosemary (*Rosmarinus officinalis* L.). Food Microbiology 11:57–63

Parke D V, Rahman H 1970 The induction of hepatic microsomal enzymes by safrole. Proceedings of the Biochemical Society 119:53–54

Parke D V, Rahman K M Q, Walker R 1974 The absorption, distribution and excretion of linalool in the rat. Biochemical Society Transactions 2:612–615

Parys B T 1983 Chemical burns resulting from contact with peppermint oil mar: a case report. Burns, Including Thermal Injury 9(5):374–375

Patel S, Wiggins J 1980 Eucalyptus oil poisoning. Archives of Disease in Childhood 55(5): 405–406

Pattnaik S, Rath C, Subramanyam V R 1995 Characterisation of resistance to essential oils in a strain of *Pseudomonas aeruginosa* (VR-6). Microbios 81:29–31

Pattnaik S, Subramanyam V R, Kole C 1996 Antibacterial and antifungal activity of ten essential oils in vitro. Microbios 86:237–246

Paumgartten F J R, Delgado I F, Alves E N, Nogueira A C, De-Farias R C, Neubert D 1990 Single dose toxicity study of beta-myrcene, a natural analgesic substance. Brazilian Journal of Medical and Biological Research 23:873–877

Pena E F 1962 *Melaleuca alternifolia* oil. Its use for trichomonas vaginitis and other vaginal infections. Obstetrics and Gynecology 19(6):793–795

Penoel D 1992 *Eucalyptus smithii* essential oil and its uses in aromatic medicine. British Journal of Phytotherapy 2(4):154–159

Penoel D 1994 Art and science. The aromatic triptych revisited. International Journal of Aromatherapy 6(3):5–7

Perez Raya M D, Utrilla M P, Navarro M C, Jimenez J 1990 CNS activity of *Mentha rotundifolia* and *Mentha longifolia* essential oil in mice and rats. Phytotherapy Research 4(6):232–234

Perfumi M, Paparelli F, Cingolani M L 1995 Spasmolytic activity of essential oil of *Artemesia thuscula* cav. from the Canary Islands. Journal of Essential Oil Research 7(4):387–392

Perruci S, Macchioni G, Cioni P C, Flamini G, Morelli I, Taccini F 1996 The activity of volatile compounds from *Lavandula angustifolia* against *Psoroptes cuniculi*. Phytotherapy Research 10(1):5–8

Piccaglia R, Deans S G, Marotti M, Eaglesham E 1993 Biological activity of essential oils from lavender, sage, winter savory and thyme of Italian origin. Programme abstracts, 24th International Symposium on Essential Oils

Pilapil V R 1989 Toxic manifestation of cinnamon oil ingestion in a child. Clinical Paediatrics 28(6):276

Price H, Lewith G, Williams C 1991 Acupressure as an anti-emetic in cancer chemotherapy. Complementary Medicine Research 5(2):93–94

Price S 1993 The aromatherapy workbook. Thorsons, Wellingborough

Puustjarvi K, Airaksinen O, Pontinen P J 1990 The effects of massage in patients with chronic tension headache. Acupuncture and Electrotherapy Research 15:159–162

Rademaker M, Kirby J D T 1987 Contact dermatitis to a skin adhesive. Contact Dermatitis 16(5):297–298

Raman A, Weir U, Bloomfield S F 1995 Antimicrobial effects of tea tree oil and its major components on *Staphylococcus aureus*, *Staph. epidermidis* and *Propionibacterium* acnes. Letters in Applied Microbiology 21:242–245

Ramanoelina A R, Terrom G P, Bianchini J P, Coulanges P 1987 Antibacterial action of essential oils extracted from Madagascar plants. Archives de l'Institut Pasteur de Madagascar 53(1):217–226 (cited in Harris B 1997 Aromatherapy Database. Essential Oil Resource Consultants, St Germain le Guillaume, France, p 17)

Rangelov A 1989 An experimental characterisation of cholagogic and cholesteric activity of a group of essential oils. Folia Medica (Plovdiv) 31(1):46–53

Rangelov A, Pisanetz M, Toreva D, Kosev R 1988 Experimental study of the cholagogic and choleretic action of some of the basic ingredients of essential oils on laboratory animals. Folia Medica (Plovdiv) 30(4):30–38

Recsan Z, Pagliuci G, Piretti M V, Penzes L G, Youdim K A, Noble R C, Deans S G 1997 Effect of essential oils on the lipids of the retina in the ageing rat: a possible therapeutic use. Journal of Essential Oil Research 9:53–56

Rees W D, Evans B K, Rhodes J 1979 Treating irritable bowel syndrome with peppermint oil. British Medical Journal 2(6194):835–836

Reynolds J E F (ed) 1993 Martindale: the extra pharmacopoeia. The Pharmaceutical Press, London

Roach B 1985 Ginger root (*Zingiber officinale*). California Association of Midwives Newsletter 1:2

Roberts A, Williams J M G 1992 The effect of olfactory stimulation on fluency, vividness of imagery and associated mood: a preliminary study. British Journal of Medical Psychology 65(2):197–199

Roffey S J, Walker R, Gibson G G 1990 Hepatic peroxisomal and microsomal induction by citral and linalool in rats. Food and Chemical Toxicology 28(6):403–408

Rompelberg C J M, Verhagen H, van Bladeren P J 1993 Effects of the naturally occurring alkenylbenzenes eugenol and *trans*-anethole on drug-metabolising enzymes in the rat liver. Food and Chemical Toxicology 31(9):637–645

Rose J E, Behm F M 1994 Inhalation of vapor from black pepper extract reduces smoking withdrawal symptoms. Drug and Alcohol Dependence 34(3):225–229

Rossi T, Melegari M, Bianchi A, Albasini A, Vampa G 1988 Sedative, anti-inflammatory and antidiuretic effects induced in rats by essential oils of varieties of *Anthemis nobilis*: a comparative study. Pharmacological Research Communications 20(suppl 5):71–74

Rothe A, Heine A, Rebohle E 1973 Oil from juniper berries as an occupational allergen for the skin and respiratory tract. Berufsdermatosen 21(1):11–16

Rubin et al 1949 Ingesting poisons – survey of 250 children. Clinical Proceedings Children's Hospital 5:57–73

Rudski E, Grzywa Z, Bruo W S 1976 Sensitivity to 35 essential oils. Contact Dermatitis 2:196–200

Ryman D 1991 Aromatherapy – the encyclopaedia of plants and oils and how they help you. Piatkus, London

Sacchetti G, Romagnoli C, Mares D, Bonsignore L, Poli F 1995 Antibacterial effects of the essential oil of *Santolina insularis* (Genn. Ex Fiori Arrig. Asteraceae). Biomedical Letters 52(207):191–195

Saeed S A, Gilani A H 1994 Antithrombotic activity of clove oil. Pakistan Medical Association 44(5):112–115

Safayhi H, Sabieraj J, Sailer E R, Ammon H P T 1994 Chamazulene: an antioxidant-type inhibitor of leucotriene B_4 formation. Planta Medica 60: 410–413

Sandbank M, Abramovici A, Wolf R, Ben David E 1988 Sebaceous gland hyperplasia following topical application of citral. American Journal of Dermatopathology 10(5):415–418

Santos F A, Rao V S N, Silveira E R 1996 Studies on the neuropharmacological effects of *Psidium guyanensis* and *Psidium pohlianum* essential oils. Phytotherapy Research 10:655–658

Santos F A, Rao V S N, Silveira E R 1997 Anti-inflammatory and analgesic activities of the essential oil of *Psidium guianense*. Fitoterapia 68(1):65–68

Schafer D, Schafer W 1981 Pharmacological studies with an ointment containing menthol, camphene and essential oils for broncholytic and secretolytic effects. Arzneimittelforschung 31(1):82–86

Schaller M, Korting H C 1995 Allergic airborne contact dermatitis from essential oils used in aromatherapy. Clinical and Experimental Dermatology 20(2):143–145

Sellar W 1992 The directory of essential oils. C W Daniel, Saffron Walden

Selvaag E, Erikson B, Thune P 1994 Contact allergy due to tea tree oil and cross-sensitisation to colophony. Contact Dermatitis 31:124–125

Selvaag E, Hol J-O, Thune P 1995 Allergic contact dermatitis in an aromatherapist with multiple sensitisations to essential oils. Contact Dermatitis 33:354–355

Seth G, Kokate C K, Varma K C 1976 Effect of essential oil of *Cymbopogon citratus* stapf. on the central nervous system. Indian Journal of Experimental Biology 14(3): 370–371

Sharma R, Bajaj A K, Singh K G 1987 Sandalwood dermatitis. International Journal of Dermatology 26(9):597

Shrivastav P, Goerge K, Balasubramaniam N et al 1988 Suppression of puerperal lactation using jasmine flowers (*Jasminum sambac*). Australian and New Zealand Journal of Obstetrics and Gynaecology 28(1):68–71

Shubina L P, Siurin S A, Savchenko V M 1990 Inhalations of essential oils in the combined treatment of patients with chronic bronchitis. Vrachebnoe Delo 5:66–67

Sims S 1986 Slow stroke back massage for cancer patients. Nursing Times 82(13):47–50

Singh G, Upadhyay R K 1991 Fingitoxic activity of cumaldehyde, main constituent of the *Cuminum cyminum* oil. Fitoterapia 62(1):86

Singh G, Upadhyay R K, Narayanan C S, Padmkumari K P, Rao G P 1993 Chemical and fungitoxic investigations on the essential oil of *Citrus sinensis* (L.) Persian Journal of Plant Diseases and Protection 100(1):69–74

Smith D G, Standing L, De Man A 1992 Verbal memory elicited by ambient odor. Perceptual and Motor Skills 74:339–343

Soliman F M, El-Kashoury E A, Fathy M M, Gonaid M H 1994 Analysis and biological activity of the essential oil of *Rosmarinus officinalis* L. from Egypt. Flavour and Fragrance Journal 9:29–33

Somerville K W, Richmond C R, Bell G D 1984 Delayed release peppermint oil capsules (Colpermin) for the spastic colon syndrome: a pharmokinetic study. British Journal of Clinical Pharmacology 18(4):638–640

Southwell I A, Markham C, Mann C 1997 Skin irritancy of tea tree oil. Journal of Essential Oil Research 9:47–52

Spoerke D G, Vandenburg S A, Smolinske S C et al 1989 Eucalyptus oils; 14 cases of exposure. Veterinary and Human Toxicology 31(2):166–168

Stanic G, Samarzija I 1993 Diuretic activity of *Satureja montana* subsp. Montana extracts and oil in rats. Phytotherapy Research 7(5):363–366

Stannard D 1989 Pressure prevents nausea. Nursing Times 85(4):33–34

Stassi V 1996 The antimicrobial activity of the essential oil of four *Juniperus* species growing wild in Greece. Flavour and Fragrance Journal 11(1):71–74

Steele J 1992 Environmental fragrancing. International Journal of Aromatherapy 4(2):9–11

Steinmetz M D, Vial M, Millet Y 1987 Actions of essential oils of rosemary and certain of its constituents (eucalyptol and camphor) on the cerebral cortex of the rat in vitro. Journal de Toxicologie Clinique et Expérimentale 7(4):259–271

Steinmetz M D, Moulin-Traffort J, Regli P 1988 Transmission and scanning electronmicroscopy study of the action of sage and rosemary essential oils and eucalyptol on *Candida albicans*. Mycoses 31(1):40–51

Stevenson C 1992 Orange blossom evaluation. International Journal of Aromatherapy 4(3):22–24

Stiles J C, Sparks M S, Ronzio B S, Ronzio R A 1995 The inhibition of *Candida albicans* by oregano. Journal of Applied Nutrition 47(4):96–102

Stimpfl T, Nasel B, Nasel C, Binder R, Vycudilik W, Buchbauer G 1995 Concentration of 1,8-cineole in human blood during prolonged inhalation. Chemical Senses 20(3):349–350

Subba M S, Soumithri T C, Suryanarayana Rao R 1967 Antimicrobial action of citrus oils. Journal of Food Science 32:225–227

Sugano H 1989 Effects of odours on mental function. Chemical Senses 14(2):303

Sugano H, Sato N 1991 Psychophysiological studies of fragrance. Chemical Senses 16(1):183–184

Sullivan S J, Williams L R, Seaborne D E, Morelli M 1991 Effects of massage on motorneuron excitability. Physical Therapy 71(8):555–560

Suresh B, Kalyanaraman V R, Dhanasekaran S, Annadurai K, Dhanaraj S A, Balasubramanian S 1995 Evaluation of santolina oil in search of new drugs against candidiasis. Indian Journal of Pharmacology 27:171–177

Suresh B, Sriram S, Dhanaraj S A, Elango K, Chinnaswamy K 1997 Anticandidal activity of *Santolina chamaecyparissus* volatile oil. Journal of Ethnopharmacology 55(2):151–159

Svoboda S G, Deans K P 1990 A study of the variability of rosemary and sage and their volatile oils on the British market: their antioxidant properties. Flavour and Fragrance Journal 7:81–87

Sweet M 1997 Alarm in hospitals over rapid spread of a nasty germ they can't destroy. Sydney Morning Herald 15.3.97

Szelenyi I, Thiemer O I K 1979 Pharmacological experiments with compounds of chamomile. III Experimental studies of the ulceroprotective effect of chamomile. Planta Medica 35:218–227

Taddei I, Giachetti D, Taddei E, Mantovani P 1988 Spasmolytic activity of peppermint, sage and rosemary essences and their major constituents. Fitoterapia 59(6):463–468

Takayama K, Nagai T 1994 Limonene and related compounds as potential skin penetration promoters. Drug Development and Industrial Pharmacy 20(4):677–684

Takeuchi S, Miyazaki Y, Yatagai M, Ide M, Kobayashi S 1991 Sensory evaluation of essential oils. Chemical Senses 16:198

Tasev T, Toleva P, Balabanova V 1969 The neuro-psychic effect of Bulgarian rose, lavender and geranium. Folia Medica (Plovdiv) 11(5):307–317

Telfer F M 1997 Relief of pain in labour. In: Sweet B R, Tiran D (eds) Mayes' midwifery, 12th edn. Baillière Tindall, London, ch 32, pp 419–434

Temple W A, Smith N A, Beasley M 1991 Management of oil of citronella poisoning. Journal of Clinical Toxicology 29(2):257–262

Tiran D, Mack S (eds) 2000 Complementary therapies for pregnancy and childbirth, 2nd edn. Baillière Tindall, London

Tisserand R 1992 The art of aromatherapy, 2nd edn. C W Daniel, Saffron Walden

Tisserand R, Balacs T 1995 Essential oil safety. A guide for health professionals. Churchill Livingstone, London

Toaff M E, Abramovici A, Sporn J, Liban E 1979 Selective oocyte degeneration and impaired fertility in rats treated with the aliphatic monoterpene Citral. Journal of Reproduction and Fertility 55:347–352

Tong M M, Altman P M, Barnetson R StC 1992 Tea tree oil in the treatment of tinea pedis. Australasian Journal of Dermatology 33(3):145–149

Trabace L, Avato P, Mazzoccoli M, Siro-Brigiani G 1992 Choleretic activity of some typical components of essential oils. Planta Medica 58(suppl 1):a650–651

Tripathi R C, Fekrat-Polascik B, Tripathi B J, Ernest J T 1990 An unusual necrotising dermatitis after a single application of topical benzoin and pressure bandage for enucleation of an eye. Lens Eye Toxic Research 7(2):173–178

Truitt E B et al 1963 Evidence of monoamine oxidase inhibition by myristicin and nutmeg. Proceedings of the Society for Experimental Biology and Medicine 112:647–650

Tubaro A, Zilli C, Redaelli C, Delia Loggia R 1984 Evaluation of anti-inflammatory activity of a chamomile extract topical application. Planta Medica 50(4):359

UK Central Council 1992a The scope of professional practice. UK Central Council, London

UK Central Council 1992b Standards for the administration of medicines. UK Central Council, London

UK Central Council 1996 Guidelines for professional practice. UK Central Council, London

UK Central Council 1998 Midwives' rules and code of practice. UK Central Council, London

Valnet J 1982 The practice of aromatherapy. C W Daniel, Saffron Walden

Van Ketel W G 1981 Allergy to *Matricaria chamomilla*. Contact Dermatitis 8(2):143

Vickers A 1997 Yes, but do we know it's true? Knowledge claims for massage and aromatherapy. Complementary Therapies in Nursing and Midwifery 3:63–65

Viollon C, Mandin D, Chaumont J P 1996 Antagonistic activities in vitro of some essential oils and natural volatile compounds in relation to the growth of *Trichomonas vaginalis*. Fitoterapia 67(3):279–280

Von Grisk A, Fischer W 1969 Pulmonary excretion of cineole, menthol and thymol in rats following rectal application. Zeitschrift für Ärztliche Fortbildung 63(4):233–236

Walding M F 1991 Pain, anxiety and powerlessness. Journal of Advanced Nursing 16:338–397

Walker P 1995 Baby massage. Piatkus, London

Walsh L J, Wagstaff J 1987 The antimicrobial effects of an essential oil on selected pathogens. Periodontology 8:11–15

Warm J S, Dember W N 1990 Effects of fragrances on vigilance performance and stress. Perfumer and Flavorist 15:15–18

Warm J S, Dember W N, Parasuraman R 1991 Effects of olfactory stimulation on performance and stress in a visual sustained attention task. Journal of the Society of Cosmetic Chemists 42:199–210

Watt M 1995 Essential oils: their lack of skin absorption but effectiveness via inhalation. The Aromatic 'Thymes' 3(2):11–33, 28

Wattenberg L W, Coccia J B 1991 Inhibition of 4-(methylnitrosamino)-1-(3-pyridyl)-1-butanone carcinogenesis in mice by *d*-limonene and citrus fruit oils. Carcinogenesis 12(1):115–117

Waymouth S 1992 Case study – essential hypertension. International Journal of Aromatherapy 4(3):29

Webb N J A, Pitt W R 1993 Eucalyptus oil poisoning in childhood: 41 cases in south-east Queensland. Journal of Paediatrics and Child Health 29:368–371

Weiss J, Catalano P 1973 Camphorated oil intoxication during pregnancy. Paediatrics 52:713–714

Weyers W, Brodbeck R 1989 Skin absorption of volatile oils. Pharmokinetics. Pharmazie in Unsere Zeit 18(3):82–86

White-Traut R C, Nelson M N 1988 Maternally administered tactile, auditory, visual and vestibular stimulation: relationship to later interactions between mothers and premature infants. Research in Nursing and Health 11:31–39

Wilkinson S 1995 Aromatherapy and massage in palliative care. International Journal of Palliative Nursing 1(1):21–30

Williams A C, Barry B W 1989 Essential oils as novel human skin penetration enhancers. International Journal of Pharmaceutics 57:R7–R9

Williams L R, Stockley J K, Yan W, Home V N 1998 Essential oils with high antimicrobial activity for therapeutic use. International Journal of Aromatherapy 8(4):30–40

Woeber K, Krombach M 1969 Sensitisation from volatile oils (preliminary report). Berufsdermatosen 17(6):320–326

Worwood V 1990 The fragrant pharmacy. Bantam Books, London

Yamada K, Mimaki Y, Sashida Y 1994 Anticonvulsive effects of inhaling lavender oil vapour. Biological and Pharmaceutical Bulletin 17(2):359–360

Yang D, Michel D, Mandin D, Andriamboavonjy H, Poitry P, Chaumont J-P 1996 Antifungal and antibacterial properties, in vitro, of three Patchouli essential oils of different origins. Acta Botanica Gallica 143(1):29–35

Yashphe J, Feuerstein I, Barel S, Segal R 1987 The antibacterial and antispasmodic activity of *Artemesia herba alba* Asso. II Examination of essential oils from various chemotypes. International Journal of Crude Drug Research 25(2):89–96

Zakarya D, Fkih-Tetouani S, Hajji F 1993 Chemical composition – antimicrobial activity relationships of Eucalyptus essential oils. Plantes Médicinales et Phytothérapie 26(4):319–331

Zangouras et al 1981 cited by Tisserand R, Balacs T 1995 *Essential Oil safety: a Guide for Health Care Professionals* Churchill Livingstone London p120

Zarno V 1994 Candidiasis. International Journal of Aromatherapy 6(2):20–23

Zarzuelo A, Navarro C, Crespo M E, Ocete M A, Jimenez J, Cabo J 1987 Spasmolytic activity of *Thymus membranaceus* essential oil. Phytotherapy Research 1(3):114–116

Zaynoun S T, Johnson B E, Frain-Bell W 1977 A study of the oil of bergamot and its importance as a phototoxic agent. British Journal of Dermatology 96:475–482

Zheng G, Kenney P M, Zhang J, Lam L K T 1992a Inhibition of benzo(*a*)pyrene-induced tumorigenesis by myristicin, a volatile aroma constituent of parsley leaf oil. Carcinogenesis 13(10):1921–1923

Zheng G Q, Kenney P M, Lam L K T 1992b Sesquiterpenes from clove (*Eugenia caryiphyllata*) as potential anticarcinogenic agents. Journal of Natural Products 55(7):999–1003

Zheng G, Kenney P, Lam K T 1993 Potential anticarcinogenic natural products isolated from lemongrass oil and galanga root oil. Journal of Agricultural and Food Chemistry 41(2):153–156

Further Reading

Ashby N 1994 Subtle anatomy and physiology. Aromatherapy Quarterly 40:29–31

Beresford-Cooke C 1995 Shiatsu theory and practice. A comprehensive textbook for student and professional. Churchill Livingstone, London

Cawthorn A 1995 A review of the literature surrounding the research into aromatherapy. Complementary Therapies in Nursing and Midwifery 1:118–120

Davies P 1997 What does the Internet offer bodyworkers? Journal of Bodywork and Movement Therapies 1(2):102–106

Ernst E (ed) 1996 Complementary medicine: an objective appraisal. Butterworth Heinemann, Oxford

Mojay G 1993 The Chinese energetic model. International Journal of Aromatherapy 5(3):9–12

Sharma U 1995 Complementary medicine today: practitioners and patients, 2nd edn. Routledge, London

Sun D 1994 The aroma of colour. Aromatherapy World, Spring 1994:21–24

Sweet B, Tiran D 1997 Mayes' midwifery, 12th edn. Baillière Tindall, London

Tiran D 1996 The use of complementary therapies in midwifery practice: a focus on reflexology. Complementary Therapies in Nursing and Midwifery 2:32–37

Tiran D, Mack S (eds) 2000 Complementary therapies for pregnancy and childbirth, 2nd edn. Baillière Tindall, London

Trevelyan J, Booth B 1995 Complementary medicine for nurses, midwives and health visitors. Macmillan, London

Vickers A 1996 Massage and aromatherapy: a guide for health professionals. Chapman & Hall, London

Wong M 1994 Do plants have souls? Exploring the esoteric properties of essential oils. Aromatherapy Quarterly 41:33–35

Websites/Database

Aromatherapy Organisations Council: http://business.virgin.net/aoc.carole/index.html

Essential Oils of India:http://members.aol.com/somanath/fragrant.html

Foundation for Integrated Medicine: http:// www.fimed.org

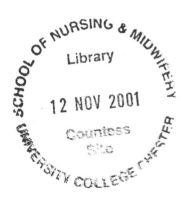

Index

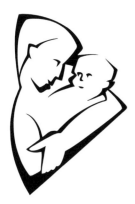

Numbers in *italics* refer to illustrations.
Numbers in **bold** refer to main reference